HOW TO FIX LYME DISEASE

3 SECRETS TO IMPROVE ANY LYME DISEASE TREATMENT

BY DR. JAY DAVIDSON

Copyright © 2017

DrJayDavidson.com

HOW TO FIX LYME DISEASE

Copyright ©2017 DrJayDavidson.com

Information provided in this book is for educational purposes only and is not intended to replace the recommendations of a qualified healthcare professional. The information in this book does not diagnose, treat, or cure any disease.

DrJayDavidson.com
5052 Clairemont Dr #17025
San Diego, California 92117
info@DrJayDavidson.com

Printed in the United States of America

First Edition (Version 1.2)

ISBN-10: 1977883435

ISBN-13: 978-1977883438

Jon N Jess Schuette with Jay Davidson in 📍 San Diego, California.
June 3 at 9:36am · 👥

The Lord turned my test into a testimony. Bedridden from Lyme disease, lost my job, friends, relationships were strained, health deteriorated to a point we didn't know if I would make it....but I stand here today with the doctor who helped me through it all at his health retreat in San Diego. Dr Jay Davidson, I owe you my life. I am now HEALTHY, LIVING, CAPABLE, and STRONGER than I've ever felt. I am proof that treating your body rather than treating the disease WORKS.

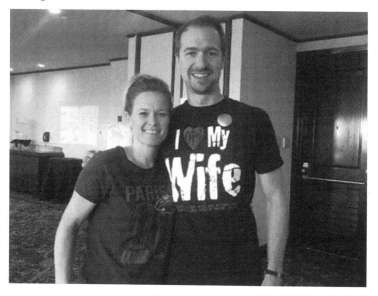

⭕ Love   💬 Comment   ➤ Share

⭕◯😊 You, JR Burgess, Chris Pellow and 185 others

OPENING THOUGHTS

A study was done by Microsoft Corp. showing that people now generally lose concentration after eight seconds. Time magazine commented that the "notoriously ill-focused goldfish is nine seconds."[1]

Since our attentions spans are quite short and with many Lyme sufferers having brain fog and memory issues, I decided to keep this book shorter.

After publishing my first book, *5 Steps to Restoring Health Protocol™*, I received many questions about how to stay updated on the most current products recommendations I have for you.

In an effort to keep you updated, I have created the following link, which will contain the most up to date products and recommendations: www.DrJayDavidson.com/FixLyme

20 WORD BOOK SUMMARY

From Mess to Message: How we healed my wife's Lyme disease and how you can learn to heal yourself too.

TABLE OF CONTENTS

INTRODUCTION

There are a variety of thoughts about Lyme disease, depending on your location, the practitioners you have worked with, and the research you have done. It dumbfounds me that there are doctors who still do not believe that Lyme disease exists. There are doctors that do not believe that "chronic" Lyme disease exists either.

On the opposite end of the spectrum, there are many doctors who do believe it exists and have dedicated their lives to giving hope to those suffering and in finding a path to healing.

For the purpose of this book, let's assume Lyme disease, specifically "chronic" Lyme disease, does exist.

There is also a vast array of different treatments and protocols out there. There is an organization called the Infectious Diseases Society of America (IDSA), which essentially only believes in short term use of antibiotics. Think of IDSA and CDC views being very similar. There is another group of doctors associated with the International Lyme and Associated Diseases Society (aka ILADS) that have written their own guidelines promoting long-term antibiotic treatment for chronic Lyme disease. There is also a third group focusing on holistic and natural herbal tools for chronic Lyme disease treatment. You generally can put a practitioner or doctor in one of the categories, or along the spectrum.

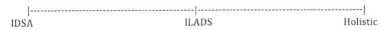

|--|--|
IDSA   ILADS   Holistic

The purpose of this book is not to convince you of THE one best treatment. If there is anything I have learned from the clients my team and I have worked with, it is that everything needs to be customized to the individual case. In this book, I aim to give you some of the best tips I have found to be game changers for those struggling with Lyme disease in their path to healing.

OBJECTIVE OF THE BOOK

The goal for this book is to show you that no matter what treatment you are doing you can implement a few simple steps to improve your treatment and protocols and subsequently speed up the healing process!

It is important to note that this book is geared towards Lyme disease; however, these principles apply across the board to improve and maintain health!

I also believe that you do not need another treatment that is supposed to cure you.

You need a coach or a guide to work with you and help put all the pieces of the puzzle together.

USE THIS BOOK AS A GUIDE and when you need further assistance, reach out to us for one on one coaching at www.DrJayDavidson.com to schedule a consult.

BEFORE WE BEGIN…

MASTER YOUR MINDSET TO MASTER YOUR HEALTH

Before we begin, I want you to close your eyes. Think about whether or not you are aware of where your mindset is. You may be fighting to keep yourself alive and restore your health but have you truly reflected on what you are fighting for? Do you know how to turn your struggles into your strengths?

There is a reason I am including mindset in the introduction. Mindset is often the pink elephant in the room and I believe it is one of the most important aspects on your path to healing. Very few are enlightened at where their mindset currently is and I want to walk you through how you can use your mindset to your advantage in this journey.

5 TIPS TO HELP IMPROVE YOUR MINDSET

1. Focus on your Big "Why"

It is important to identify your "WHY." What are your passions in life? What activities make you happy? Who do you live for (HINT: Part of this answer should always include yourself)? What is your purpose in life? When we answer these questions, we can focus our mindset on these vital pieces of our life.

One of the main aspects that got my wife through her near death experience was her love for Leela and wanting to be around for her as she grew up.

2. Identify Unrealistic Expectations

We all have unrealistic expectations at one point or another. It is important to take time to mentally explore events, actions or feelings that you have experienced negatively in the past. Often times, unmet expectations simply equal frustration and resentment, which ultimately gets us nowhere and fills us with negative thoughts and feelings. By understanding that you cannot control the behavior of others, and changing your expectations accordingly, you can start focusing on yourself and your own healing instead.

The chances that one magic idea or thing is going to heal you at 100% within a matter of a few short weeks would fit into this category. There are certainly helpful tools that can improve how you are feeling and your case, however, it is important to put all of the pieces of the puzzle together, and in the right order, to heal the body. Working with a personal coach who can guide you on your journey to restoring your health is vitally important. This is important to not only coach you to get well, but also to teach you how to take care of yourself and ensure you do not end back up where you are or were.

3. Turn your Struggles into your Strengths

In the words of American author Byron Katie: *"Life is simple. Everything happens for you, not to you. Everything happens at exactly the right moment, neither too soon nor too late. You don't have to like it...it's just easier if you do."* It is easy to feel like the world is against you when in a seemingly endless pit of hardship and frustration; whether it be through chronic illness or something else you are going through in life. It is important to remember that for every difficult situation you go through, you have the ability to learn valuable life lessons and turn them into your strengths moving forward.

Each moment of Heather's struggles was hard on both her and our family, however, we would never be where we are now without the opportunity to learn from each and every one of the hardships we have been through.

4. Attitude of Gratitude

Gratitude has been linked to greater health and happiness. As we go through struggles in life, especially when ourselves or someone close to us is faced with a life threatening illness, it can make us take a step back and reflect on what we have. Even if we have things in life that we have not taken for granted, we may not have appreciated them as much as we should have in the past. Cultivating gratitude can have a profound impact on our mindset and, in turn, our ability to heal. To practice gratitude, try keeping a daily gratitude journal. You can ask yourself

"Who or what inspired me today?", "What brought me happiness today?", and "What brought me comfort and deep peace today?" Alternatively, you could take 15-20 minutes out of each day to sit quietly or take a walk and reflect. As you do so, consider the things in which you are grateful for: relationships, your body, your mind, nature, and even material comforts. It is important to realize the abundance in your life and focus on the things that fill your soul with happiness and gratitude.

5. Forgive and Release

Holding resentment and anger inside of us can cloud our thoughts and limit our ability for a healing mindset. Forgiveness does not mean rationalizing bad behavior or forgetting what might have happened that was hurtful for you. The most important part of forgiveness is realizing that you are not doing it for someone else; you are doing it for YOU. Once you have experienced true forgiveness by releasing it, you will realize that although we cannot predict what will happen in life, we always have the ability to choose how we respond to it.

The key word here is "release." Once you do this, you can create space in your mind to focus on what is important to move you forward in healing. Yes, there are times we need to vent, but if all you speak is complaining, you immediately shut down your creativity to fix or see other solutions to what is going on.

Stop complaining about a label you were given and took on and create a roadmap to heal.

Stop complaining about not having any money for treatment and create an environment that can produce what you need.

Stop complaining about the things you view as negative and start creating a list of what you are grateful for in your life.

This idea that you will be happy only when you get well is foolish. YOU have the ability inside of you to decide to be happy today! To create an environment where you can focus on the positive and eliminate negativity.

Create happiness for yourself today and avoid complaining.

Chapter 1. Our Story

Chronic Lyme Disease Healed After 25 Years

My wife Heather is the reason I have dedicated my life to helping others heal from Lyme disease. I became an expert not because of my professional schooling, or even my desire to become successful. I learned these principles because I wanted to save my wife. My journey began in darkness as I faced the reality of my wife's deteriorating condition and the inability to find doctors who could offer her any relief.

Heather's health history is complicated, as with most cases of Lyme disease. She first became ill when she was seven years old. Despite visiting many doctors and running countless tests, nothing came back with conclusive results. She was prescribed various medications, even though no one really knew what she was being treated for. Not long after she began these medications, she suddenly ended up with encephalitis (brain swelling) and went into a coma for six weeks. After finally discovering she was suffering from Lyme disease, she was given intravenous (IV) antibiotics and soon awoke from her comatose state. The antibiotics were enough to keep her functioning but did not fix the source. Throughout her childhood, various health problems continued to appear and wreak havoc on her life. One of her most painful memories is of the time she was unable to compete in the Junior Olympics due to unexplained sinus issues that caused her to be unable to breathe. Unfortunately, she continued to struggle like this all throughout her childhood, just barely getting by.

Then, the symptoms of her Lyme disease began to appear in full force again when she was 18 years old. The disease never really left her system; it had just been "dulled" for a few years. On one occasion, she fell to the floor and almost passed out. While being taken to the hospital by ambulance, the EMTs discovered she had a resting heart rate of 260 beats per minute. A normal range for an adult is 60-100 beats per minute. She was diagnosed with supraventricular tachycardia (SVT), a condition that caused her heart to beat out of control and would lead to two heart surgeries.

Problem after problem kept popping up and her physical condition was getting worse. The trauma associated with dealing with a chronic illness, and especially not being able find the answers she was looking for, caused deep emotional distress and frustration.

Heather and I met in 2004 at a time when she was doing "okay" and in another phase of her life we term as "just getting by." She would do "okay" for a while, then we would deal with health crash after health crash. We would scramble and try to keep things from getting worse. When the "storm" would leave, we were back to just keeping the boat afloat.

On Heather's 30th birthday, after 25 hours of labor, she gave birth to our beautiful daughter Leela.

The pregnancy was hard on Heather and it really took its toll. I certainly developed a whole new respect for mothers going through the pregnancy and birthing process. I am truly amazed at how tough women are.

After Leela was born, Heather's health continued to deteriorate and her body was just not able to heal itself. It took about six months before Heather could even walk normal. When Leela was two months old, it was the absolute bottom for Heather and she had to stop breastfeeding since her body was not able to handle it.

At that point Heather stopped being able to eat anything. Everything she ate or drank other than traditional bone broth or water would cause her throat to swell up and shut her down. For 17 days, she was only able to consume bone broth and water and subsequently lost 50 pounds. On day 18, she was finally able to slowly add in solid foods again, increasing slowly as time went on.

Her fatigue and frustration was slow to turn around. We went through it all as we searched for a remedy: sleepless nights, fights between us over nothing, and overwhelming feelings of frustration and fear. Even though we are both doctors, we were puzzled and left with a seemingly endless list of problems that appeared to have no solutions. This led to a desperate quest with countless of hours researching for anything and anyone that could possibly help us.

I vividly remember countless nights lying in bed next to my wife, not being able to fall asleep as I worried about the possibility that she would not wake up in the morning. I was not willing to lose my wife, my best friend, and the mother of our newborn daughter. I still get tears in my eyes re-living those feelings.

It felt like a tailspin and I remember having thoughts about whether our daughter was a curse to us. I feel so regretful for those thoughts as we know she was such an incredible blessing for Heather and I. If it were not for Leela being born into this world, Heather most likely would have never been forced to go upstream and find out the root cause of her health issues in the first place. I believe it was her love for Leela that gave her the drive and courage to take on what felt like an unbeatable giant.

A list of the symptoms and conditions my wife had:

- Insomnia
- Temperature dysregulation
- Hormonal dysfunction
- Supraventricular tachycardia (requiring two heart surgeries)
- Vertigo and dizziness
- Chronic sinus infections (requiring sinus scraping surgery)
- Reproductive issues

- Leaky gut
- Acid reflux
- Constipation
- Adrenal fatigue
- Mold toxicity
- Multiple chemical sensitivities
- Brain fog (memory and concentration problems)
- Migraine headaches
- Severe joint pain
- Carpal tunnel
- Mycoplasma
- Anxiety
- Chronic Lyme disease (for twenty-five years)
- *Bartonella*, *Babesia*
- Epstein-Barr virus
- Mercury and lead heavy metal toxicity
- Autoimmune thyroid
- Asthma
- Shortness of breath
- Chest pain
- Fibromyalgia
- Brain encephalitis
- Severe allergies
- Costochondritis
- Myositis ossificans (requiring surgery)
- Liver problems (causing jaundice)
- Diastasis recti (that created extreme pain in her pelvic floor and vaginal area)
- Painful gallbladder attacks

- Whiplash from multiple car accidents
- *Helicobacter pylori*

Think of Heather as the canary in a coal mine. If there is something wrong in the atmosphere, she is always the first to know. In the past, she would suffer for days after being exposed to a moldy building. Cologne or perfume would instantly give her a headache and leave her with brain fog (*more on that later*). Needless to say, this limited the places she was able to go. We could never even think about going into a store with fragrances or candles, let alone even walk by one in a shopping mall.

She was a severely sick and sensitive person. I was so frustrated as I had treated people in this condition in the past and had successfully helped them to renewed wellness. With Heather it was different: if a treatment worked for someone else, it did not work for her and usually made things worse!

We reached out for help, a lot of help. In fact, we spent over $110,000 on appointments, treatments and devices from anyone or anything we thought would help cure her. Along with the funds we spent on doctors and treatments, we spent over $400,000 for education and seminars. All in all, the quest for a cure added up to well over $500,000.

It's safe to say that Heather thought about throwing in the towel many times out of frustration and desperation. This was where I was able to give her the help and support I so desperately wanted to provide. I am relentless, persistent, and intense. I refused to give up and knew that the answers we were looking for had to be out there. *They had to be.*

No one has ever grown on top of the mountain. Don't get me wrong, it feels great to be on top of the mountain, but it is in the valleys that we grow. When it feels like your world is crashing in on you, you are suddenly willing to step outside of your comfort zone and reach beyond what you thought you could achieve.

Despite all of this, neither of us were willing to give up! There were definitely a lot of tough moments, but we never lost hope that we would find the solution we were looking for. We just didn't know *when, how,* or even *what* it would be.

WHEN PEOPLE READ OR HEAR ABOUT MY WIFE'S STORY TODAY, THE MOST COMMON QUESTION I GET IS: "HOW IS SHE DOING NOW?"

I am happy to report that she is the healthiest she has ever been! She is vibrant, strong and glowing as an amazing woman!

She used to get extremely winded doing any activity. That's gone.

She use to have horrible brain fog and couldn't remember much detail or past daily activities. I am happy to report that she has surpassed my photographic memory!

We tackled every single one of her symptoms and she is now able to live active, fulfilling life.

CHAPTER 2. LYME FACTS AND INFORMATION

Lyme disease deserves credit for being spread by many vectors, being misunderstood and often times difficult to diagnose, and for being extremely tough to kill. My team and I created a video called "All about Lyme Disease in under 200 seconds." You can find the video on Facebook and YouTube. The video went viral on Facebook getting over 200,000 views within two weeks. I encourage you to check it out.

Let's talk facts about Lyme disease.
If you are the analytical type, you will appreciate this chapter.

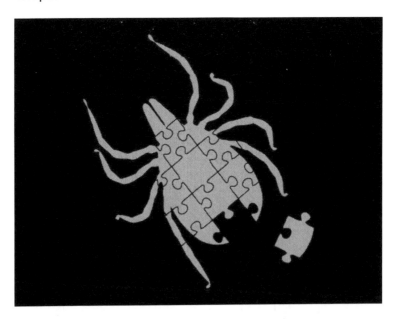

*DEPENDING ON **WHOM** YOU ARE COMMUNICATING*

WITH ABOUT LYME DISEASE, THE TOPIC CAN GET HEATED. HERE IS SOME HOUSEKEEPING KNOWLEDGE.

Lyme disease is a proper name, which means the "L" in Lyme is capitalized and the "d" for disease is not.

There is no "s" on the end of Lyme.

Lyme disease awareness month is in May.

Lyme disease has no relationship with the lime fruit other than a "Lime Challenge" for Lyme disease.

Lyme disease is a bacteria. The most widely known type is *Borrelia burgdorferi*. There have also been other types that cause Lyme disease such as *Borrelia miyamotoi* and *Borrelia mayonii*. The prestigious Mayo Clinic, who previously didn't recognize Lyme disease, discovered *Borrelia mayonii* and changed their tune.

There are over 100 strains of *Borrelia* in the USA and over 300 different strains across the world.

Lyme disease has four forms: spirochete, cyst/round body, intracellular and biofilm.

It was previously believed that one of the forms was a cell wall deficient form. Science is now showing that was an inaccurate term for the Lyme bacteria.[2]

Lyme disease is classically known to be spread via a tick called the *Ixodes scapularis*. There are other ticks that deserve attention too such as the *Ixodes pacificus*. Lyme disease has been found in lone star ticks (*Amblyomma americanum*) and gulf coast ticks (*Amblyomma maculatum*).[3] Dog ticks (Dermacentor variabilis).[4]

I Can't Get Lyme Disease if the tick was attached less than 24 hours: FALSE!

Most research on tick transmission times were performed on animals with long fur, which would require more travel time for the tick to get to the skin. A tick attached for even a short time period can transmit Lyme disease to the body.[5, 6]

The only way to get Lyme disease is via a tick bite (technically a sting): FALSE!

Most individuals that contract Lyme disease don't get it from a tick bite.

Mites, fleas, mosquitoes and biting flies can transmit Lyme disease. [7, 8, 9, 10, 11, 12, 13, 14, 15, 16, 17, 18, 19, 20, 21, 22, 23] Deer, birds, cows, rabbits, other mammals, and rodents can also be carriers of Lyme.[21, 24, 25]

Lyme disease can be spread through sex.[26] It also is found in semen samples.[27, 28] Mom's can pass it onto babies in the womb.[29] Mom's can pass *Babesia* onto child.[30] Mom's can pass on *Bartonella* onto child.[31] Animals, such as cows, have shown to have Lyme disease in the milk which would make sense that mother's could pass Lyme disease to baby via breast

18

milk.[24]

Lyme bacteria survives in human blood stored at blood banks.[32] Lyme disease can be contracted via dead fragments of the spirochete.[33] Lyme can be transmitted via urine.[34]

You have to get a bull's eye rash in order to contract Lyme disease: FALSE!

Most cases do not develop a bull's eye rash. Only 30% of those infected with Lyme disease will develop a bull's eye rash.[35, 36] Remember there are four different forms of the Lyme bacteria. If the Lyme bacteria is not in a spirochete form during transmission, there will be no bull's-eye rash.

I don't live in area that has Lyme disease: FALSE!

While there are definitely hot spots around the USA and globe. Lyme disease has been found on every continent in the world except Antarctica. Experts like Dr. Ray Strickler say that migratory birds are a big contributor to the worldwide spread of Lyme disease.[37]

Lyme disease is not an epidemic: FALSE!

In 2013, the CDC conservatively estimated that 300,000 Americans contract Lyme disease each year. Before 2013, they had previously stated that 30,000 people contract Lyme disease each year. Some experts believe that the actual number is 10x the newest CDC number. Using the 300,000 Lyme disease number makes it more common than breast cancer![38]

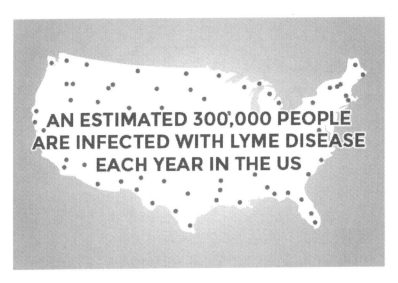

Lyme disease is not expensive: FALSE!

Tell that to someone who has been to 30 doctors, is still looking for answers and has massive relationship issues. Lyme disease not only can be monetarily costly but also typically is most costly with personal relationships, including someone's social circle. According to an unpublished school study by the CDC, the median duration of an episode of Lyme disease is 363 days at an average cost of about $100,000 per patient.[34]

What test is best to diagnose Lyme disease?

Lyme disease is a clinical diagnosis, which means the doctor uses multiple tools and resources for diagnosis, not just relying on what a test result says.

This is an important concept to understand, We do not ever want to rely on one thing as the definitive answer for being diagnosed, or to rely on one tool that is going to be a magic "cure" to get us well.

It is important to think of lab tests as a tool, examination as a tool going through someone's history as a tool, and energetic testing as a tool. I believe they all have a place, but none of these are a stand-alone tool that will fix everything.

That being said, I recommended the iSpot Lyme test by Pharmasen Labs in my last book. It was a pivotal test to help bring clarification to my wife and what was going on with her when the bottom fell out and she was extremely sick. That recommendation became outdated pretty quickly. I won't get into why as much as say the clinical world can change very rapidly as we learn more and more what is working and what is not.

If I run a laboratory test on a client for Lyme disease, currently at the time of this publication, I will use the Lyme panel by DNA Connexions in Colorado. It is a urine test that you can order without a doctor. It is not 100% accurate as no lab test is, but it is currently my top choice. It will not only check four different genes found on *Borrelia burgdorferi*, but will also check for *Borrelia miyamotoi* and *Borrelia recurrentis*. In addition, it checks for some the following coinfections: *Babesia, Bartonella, Ehrlichia* and anaplasmosis.

BEWARE OF STANDARD LYME TESTING

Standard Lyme disease testing involves a 2-tier method of the ELISA test and the Western Blot test. The ELISA test has to come back positive in order for most doctors to approve a Western Blot test. Research shows that 50-70% of patients go undiagnosed or are misdiagnosed due to the low sensitivity of traditional antibody-based testing.[39]

WHAT ARE THE SYMPTOMS OF LYME DISEASE?

Lyme is called the "The New Great Imitator"

Lyme disease has over 150 possible different symptoms associated with it

And will vary its presentation among each person too!

Symptoms, according to Global Lyme Alliance, include:

- Headache
- Facial paralysis
- Tingling in the face
- Stiff neck
- Sore throat
- Swollen glands
- Heightened allergies
- Muscle twitching
- Jaw pain
- Change in smell or taste
- Upset stomach (nausea, vomiting)

- Irritable bladder
- Unexplained weight loss or gain
- Loss of appetite, anorexia
- Difficulty breathing
- Night sweats or unexplained chills
- Heart palpitations
- Diminished exercise tolerance
- Heart block, murmur
- Chest pain or rib soreness
- Mood swings, irritability, agitation
- Depression and anxiety
- Personality changes
- Impulsive aggressive behavior
- Suicidal thoughts
- Overemotional reactions
- Disturbed sleep
- Paranoia and/or hallucinations
- Feeling as though you are losing your mind
- Obsessive-compulsive behavior
- Bipolar manic behavior
- Schizophrenic-like, including hallucinations
- Dementia
- Forgetfulness, memory loss
- Attention or concentration issues
- Confusion
- Getting lost or feeling lost

Females:

- Unexplained menstrual pain, irregularity

- Reproduction problems, miscarriage, stillbirth, premature birth
- Extreme PMS symptoms
- Pelvic pain
- Double or blurry vision
- Wandering or lazy eye
- Pink eye
- Sensitivity to light
- Eye pain or swelling
- Eye floaters
- Decreased hearing
- Ringing or buzzing in ears
- Sound sensitivity
- Pain in ears
- Joint pain, swelling, or stiffness
- Pain moving
- Muscle pain or cramps
- Poor muscle coordination, loss of reflexes
- Loss of muscle tone, muscle weakness

Neurologic System:
- Numbness in body, tingling, pinpricks
- Burning sensations in the body
- Burning in feet
- Weakness or paralysis of limbs
- Tremors or unexplained shaking
- Seizures, stroke
- Poor balance, dizziness, difficulty walking
- Increased motion sickness

- Lightheadedness, fainting
- Encephalopathy (cognitive impairment from brain involvement)
- Encephalitis (inflammation of the brain)
- Meningitis (inflammation of the protective membrane around the brain)
- Encephalomyelitis (inflammation of the brain and spinal cord)
- Academic or vocational decline
- Difficulty with multitasking
- Difficulty with organization and planning
- Auditory processing problems
- Word finding problems
- Slowed speed of processing

Skin Problems:

- Benign tumor-like nodules
- Erythema migrans (rash)

General Well-being:

- Decreased interest in play (children)
- Extreme fatigue, tiredness, exhaustion
- Unexplained fevers (high or low grade)
- Flu-like symptoms (early in the illness)
- Symptoms seem to change, come and go

Other Organ Problems:

- Dysfunction of the thyroid (under or over active thyroid glands)
- Liver inflammation

- Bladder & kidney problems (including bed wetting)

And consider Lyme if you have ever been diagnosed with the following:

- Autoimmune condition
- Fibromyalgia
- Lupus
- Chronic fatigue syndrome (CFS)
- Depression
- Rheumatoid arthritis (RA)
- ALS
- Mental illness
- ADHD
- Multiple sclerosis (MS)
- Hypochondria
- Migraine headaches
- Anxiety
- Insomnia
- Food allergies
- Parkinson's disease
- Alzheimer's disease
- Tourette's syndrome

LYME DISEASE HISTORY

The *Borrelia burgdorferi* bacteria has been found in a 5,300-year-old ice mummy dubbed Ötzi.

In 1883, Europe documented Lyme disease in The Fitzpatrick's Dermatology in General Medicine

At that time, it was called "erythema chronicum migrans".

1902, Karl Herxheimer and Kuno Hartmann called it ACA (acrodermatitis chronica atrophicans) or Bannwarth syndrome.

1909, Arvin Afzelius of Sweden, called the rash a migrating rash erythema chronicum migrans (later shortened to erythema migrans or EM) and he suggested it came from a tick bite.

In 1930, Sven Hellerstrom identified a peculiar rash with CNS disease that caused meningitis & encephalitis. He stepped up the prediction and thought it came from a spiral-shaped bacterium, a spirochete, transmitted by ticks.

In 1965, Dr. Sidney Robbin, a semiretired internist living in Montauk, New York, described expanding circular rashes that appeared in conjunction with a peculiar type of arthritis that he named Montauk knee.

In 1968, a Wisconsin dermatologist, noted what appears to be Lyme disease from a 57-year-old physician that went hunting in northern Wisconsin.

A bunch of kids and grown ups in Lyme, Connecticut, in the early 70's: suffered with mysterious and debilitating issues. This is where the word Lyme came from.

In 1981, Willy Burgdorfer discovered that a bacterium

called a spirochete, carried by ticks, was causing Lyme disease. This is where the scientific name *burgdorferi* comes from.

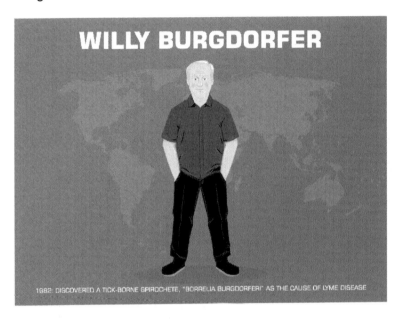

WILLY BURGDORFER

1982: DISCOVERED A TICK-BORNE SPIROCHETE, "BORRELIA BURGDORFERI" AS THE CAUSE OF LYME DISEASE

WHAT WOULD I DO IF I GOT A TICK BITE (TECHNICALLY A STING)?

How to Safely Remove a Tick and Prevent Lyme Disease

Step 1 – Remove tick properly!

Use a tick removal device to SPIN the tick and pull. Avoid tweezers if you can. DO NOT put anything on the tick including essential oils (especially peppermint oil), alcohol, flame, etc.

Step 2 – Put anti-spirochete essential oil over bite mark

Use essential oils ONLY after tick has been removed on skin such as wormseed oil.

Step 3 – Take ledum palustre 200c homeopathic (or 30c if you cannot find 200c)

This is taken every three hours for the first day, followed by twice daily for a week. This is then used twice weekly for a month and then once per week for another month.

I recommend that everyone have these supplies on hand now. That way you will be prepared in case you or a loved one gets a tick sting.

Celebrities that have been affected by Lyme disease:

- Jennifer Capriati (Tennis Hall of Fame)
- George W. Bush
- Alec Baldwin
- Richard Gere
- Ben Stiller
- Christy Turlington (supermodel)
- Jamie-Lynn Sigher (Sopranos actress)
- Ashley Olsen
- Debbie Gibson
- Steven Colter (Flow Guy)
- Yolanda Foster (Housewives of Beverly Hills)
- Daryl Hall (Hall and Oates Band)
- Karen Allen (Indiana Jones Female Star)
- Avril Lavigne

LYME DISEASE COINFECTIONS

Myth – You only have Lyme! Often there are many other pathogens along with Lyme disease.[40, 41] The more symptoms you have the more likely you are to have co-infections. The six most common coinfections are *Babesia*, *Bartonella*, *Ehrlichia*, mycoplasma, Rocky Mountain Spotted Fever and Epstein-Barr virus.

Babesia is a malaria-like blood parasite with some bacteria like properties as well that can change its outer surface proteins and evade the immune system. *Babesia* classically causes night sweats, headaches, shortness of breath (aka air hunger), chills, fever, fatigue, the inability to maintain your weight, and muscle and joint pain.[42]

Cucurmin is a powerful anti-inflammatory herb that has antimalarial compounds which have been demonstrated to be effective against *Babesia*.[43] Artemisinin has been known to be quite effective against malaria and is a fantastic herb for *Babesia*. Research also shows that it's a great tool for *Leishmania*, *Trypanosoma*, *Toxoplamsa gondii*, *Cryptosporidium parvum*, *Giardia*, and others.[44] Clinically if you have night sweats, heart palpitations or heart flipping and/or shortness of breath (aka air hunger), think *Babesia*![45]

Bartonella is a bacterial infection that targets the central nervous system and brain. It usually presents itself with a rash or papule (a small, red, raised bump on the skin) that progresses until it becomes blistery or crusty. *Bartonella* also causes lymph nodes to swell in 1 to 2 weeks after infection. Symptoms include seizures, ophthalmological problems, sarcoidosis (inflammation of lymph nodes), brain encephalitis and even stretch marks.[43] *Bartonella* is the primary cause of "cat scratch disease" and is easily transmitted by fleas, sandflies, lice, ticks, mosquitos, midges, chiggers, biting flies, scabies, and mites. This bacteria is slow growing and takes about 24 hours to double in number. The bacteria accumulate in red blood cells, the spleen, the liver, and in bone marrow. The erythrocyte sedimentation rate is also often elevated.[42] While Lyme disease by itself alters mood and can cause depression, most psychiatric symptoms infected people suffer from are related to *Bartonella*.[46]

I believe my wife when she was 7 years old with brain encephalitis had Bartonella and that she most likely contracted it from her cat. She still has many cat scratch scars on her skin from when she was younger. This along with parasites is the reason that I would be very cautious having a cat or dog as a pet.

Ehrlichia is a bacterial infection that typically causes a high fever, severe headaches, flulike symptoms, muscle pains, abdominal pain, jaundice, and fatigue. Blood shown to contain *Ehrlichia* can have a low white blood cell count (leukopenia), low platelet count (thrombocytopenia), and elevated liver function (AST, ALT).[43]

Mycoplasma is larger than a virus, but smaller than typical bacteria. In fact, they are the smallest self-replicating life form known to man.[47] They are so small that 4,000 mycoplasma bacteria can fit inside one red blood cell! Mycoplasma is one of the main causes of rheumatoid arthritis and can be transmitted through insect bites, small open wounds, inhalation, ingestion, and sex. It also causes pneumonia and has even been linked to Tourette's syndrome. Research shows that a mycoplasma infection is very common in ALS patients (amyotrophic lateral sclerosis).[42]

Walking pneumonia or Gulf War syndrome is actually a mycoplasma infection. People who are infected with mycoplasma often experience an increase of their symptoms when the atmospheric pressure changes. Mycoplasma provokes autoimmune issues too.

One the most obvious symptoms is sporadic sleep and the nights you get a good nights sleep, you don't feel rested. It also can make you feel completely wiped out with absolutely no energy. Mycoplasma loves cholesterol and preformed sterols. Some believe mycoplasma is a man made bacteria.

Magnesium deficiency is always an issue for people suffering from a mycoplasma infection. I recommend that clients with these issues take a magnesium supplement and avoid arginine.

Rocky Mountain Spotted Fever (RMSF) is caused by the bacteria called *Rickettsia rickettsia*. Symptoms include a sudden fever, maculopapular rash on soles of hands and feet that spreads over the entire body. Also could include headaches and bleeding issues.

Epstein-Barr virus research has shown that up to 95% of the population across the world today may be infected with the Epstein-Barr virus, or EBV – which can be found within the herpes family.[48] Within its acute and highly-infectious stage, the disease can be transmitted through bodily secretions such as saliva and genital fluids, and there have been some links between tick-transmitted diseases and EBV too.

A stealthy virus – EBV uses DNA methylation to hide from the immune system and stays within the resting memory B cells. Because these cells change along with the immune system, they protect the pathogen, and allow the EBV virus to proliferate without being detected.

Similarly to many of the viruses associated with tick-transmitted pathogens, including Lyme disease, the symptoms of EBV can include:

- Spleen enlargement
- Swollen lymph nodes
- Sore throat
- Fever
- Fatigue

Some patients also experience episodes of jaundice, which my wife had for years.[49]

CHAPTER 3. SECRET #1 DRAINAGE

WHAT IS DRAINAGE?

Drainage refers to the body's normal pathways of excreting and moving waste products out of the body. Drainage pathways would include the colon, kidneys, liver/bile duct system, the body lymphatic system, the brain lymphatic system (often referred to as the glymphatic system) and the skin.

If you have health issues, I can pretty much guarantee that your drainage pathways need to be improved. A common reason Lyme disease sufferers get symptoms with treatment of killing Lyme and/or detoxification is that the drainage pathways are not optimal. When these pathways are not open, they cannot drain the debris from the pathogens and/or cannot drain the toxins that are being pulled out of the body.

I love to use the word drainage instead of detox, as it seems there are many different meanings and interpretations for the word detox.

I personally think of "detox" as the pulling of chemicals or toxins out of the body such as mercury, lead, glyphosate, etc. I like using the word drainage to refer to the normal pathways that the body uses to move fluids around and out of the body.

USING DRAINAGE IN HEALING

"Drainage" is something that I can credit to helping some of the absolute toughest cases I have worked on. When working through protocols for healing, it is important to look "upstream" and find the source, or sources, that are preventing the body from functioning properly. I have found drainage to be an issue in every single case I have worked with. By working through various protocols, each one of these clients has been able to restore proper functioning.

For the purposes of this book, let's focus on the most important drainage area of the body: The liver and bile duct system.

The liver is the detox lifeline of the body. The liver is responsible for phase one and phase two detoxification, and is what I believe to be the most underappreciated and often overlooked organ in the body. The bile duct system is responsible for phase 3 detoxification.

The area to highlight here is what happens with those toxins once they have been processed in the liver through phase one and two detoxification. There is a third phase of detoxification, which actually has nothing to do with detoxing, but rather the excretion of toxins the body has processed. Phase three detox essentially is how the liver eliminates those toxins.

The liver manufacturers bile and about 80% of the toxins are dumped into the bile after the liver

36

processes them. The bile has two main purposes: neutralizing the stomach acid that gets released into the small intestine from the stomach (so the acid doesn't burn holes in the intestinal lining) and emulsifying the fat from the food we eat.

The bile is produced by the liver and is stored in the gallbladder sack. If someone has had their gallbladder out, this is usually a sign of massive bile duct flow issues. Unfortunately, taking the gallbladder out, does not fix the underlying issues! If anything, it can make it tougher for the body to get well and continue to function normally.

The stomach also plays an important role in the body's drainage system. It is well documented in the literature that the body needs proper stomach acid to digest food. Therefore, functional medicine practitioners often recommend things that help to improve stomach acid such as betaine HCl or consuming 1-2 tbsp. of apple cider vinegar in 8 ounces of water 30 minutes before a meal.

Those tools can help increase stomach in the short term, but will not fix the problem long term. Instead of solely treating the symptom of low stomach acid, it is important to ask is WHY there is low stomach acid in the first place.

In most cases I have worked with, the reason for low stomach acid has been because of IMPROPER BILE FLOW. When there is improper bile flow, the body is not able to produce an adequate amount of bile to neutralize the stomach acid. The body then reduces stomach acid, as it believes it is making too much. Since the body is purposefully decreasing the acid due to inadequate bile flow, giving something to increase stomach acid is not necessarily the solution.

The solution in my mind is to improve the bile flow which than will allow the body to increase stomach acid back to the proper amount. Low stomach acid is a gateway to allowing parasites, viruses, bacteria and other invaders to enter the body. Having the proper amount of stomach acid is a first line of defense to shielding these pathogens, which is why acid reflux medications that decrease stomach acid are referred to as a gateway drug.

WHY LIVER BILE DUCT?

You may be wondering why I believe the liver bile duct is the most important drainage area of the body. First and foremost, it is important to understand that the lymphatic system has twice as much fluid as the cardiovascular system! The lymphatic system is an interconnected network of organs and tissues that help to rid the body of waste and toxins. The primary function of this system is to transport lymph, a fluid that contains infection-fighting blood cells around the body.

It might be easier to think of the lymphatic system as the body's drainage system, as it works alongside other organs like your liver to clean up and dispose of waste that is left around within your body. A healthy lymphatic system also:

- Drains fluid back into the bloodstream to avoid excess swelling and inflammation.
- Filters lymph nodes to limit the way toxins spread in the body.
- Filters the blood, removing old cells and replacing them with new ones.
- Removes impurities from the body, using the liver and bladder to cleanse the system of unwanted substances, while maintaining useful substances like nutrients and vitamins.
- Fights infection with the use of special white blood cells that produce antibodies – responsible for fighting back against disease.

The lymphatic system DEPENDS on the liver bile duct drainage system in order for lymphatic drainage to occur. Additionally, the brain glymphatic system depends on the drainage of the body lymphatic system in order to clear fluids from it as well.

Simply stated, if the liver bile duct drainage pathways are clogged, then the body lymphatic drainage is clogged, and in turn, the brain glymphatic drainage is also clogged. They both depend on the liver bile duct system in order to function properly.

In working with clients to improve the liver bile duct flow, I have seen that often times it will help with constipation symptoms as well since constipation is also a drainage issue.

DRAINAGE AND LYME DISEASE

Lyme disease can contribute to the lymphatic system being clogged up, as there is evidence to show that Lyme disease likes to live in the lymphatic system.[50]

Stagnation is Lyme disease's best friend, as pathogens love to cause stagnation in the body. In order to function properly, the body requires movement or motion. You have probably heard of the phrase "motion is life", often in the exercise world, but this concept also applies to the drainage system of the body. The body needs movement to keep it functioning optimally and to create an environment that is not favorable for the pathogens, such as Lyme, to live in.

SUGGESTIONS FOR IMPROVEMENT OF DRAINAGE

Now that you have a basic foundation to understanding the drainage pathways and liver bile duct system, you may be wondering what you can do to improve upon them.

Tauroursodeoxycholic Acid or "TUDCA"

My wife will tell you that I am known to go down rabbit holes researching things she has no idea why or how I came to certain topics. I don't quite know either sometimes, but I go with it. During one of those moments, I started researching what steroid users in the bodybuilding world might do to protect their liver from damage. During my intensive research, I came across something called TUDCA.

TUDCA, otherwise known as tauroursodeoxycholic acid, is well known in the weight lifting world. Due to its immense benefits, my goal is to help bring it into the functional medicine world.

As a water-soluble bile acid, this substance has shown significant potency in treating issues with bile backup in the liver. It also can counteract the toxicity of typical bile acids, rehabilitate the liver after exposure to dangerous chemicals, and generally defend cells.

The reason that TUDCA has been so popular among bodybuilders is that it helps to protect and repair the liver after it has been exposed to the damaging impact of anabolic steroids. TUDCA is not just designed for people who are focused on building bigger muscles. The truth is that this substance, at its core, is a beneficial organ cleanser that can assist the liver bile duct system in ways I have not seen with any other product.

It is important to note that TUDCA could be beneficial in treating other conditions that have an impact on the liver bile duct system, such as Lyme disease. After all, if this substance can help to cleanse and detoxify the system, it may also be able to help with the symptoms of Lyme disease and even reduce a person's chances of suffering from chronic infections.

HOW TUDCA HELPS THE LIVER

As mentioned, TUDCA is a water-soluble bile acid that can be found naturally occurring within the human body. Despite internet rumors of where supplemental TUDCA comes from, the TUDCA that I recommend is extracted from plants and vegetables. It is renowned as one of the most powerful liver-protection substances on the market and has a fantastic ability to counteract the toxicity of regular bile acids while cleansing the liver and protecting lymphatic cells.[51]

There is some evidence that TUDCA can be beneficial for other areas throughout the body in addition to the liver. For instance, it may be able to reduce stress within a cell's Endoplasmic Reticulum, helping with insulin resistance and diabetes.[52] However, liver cleansing and protection are considered to be its primary benefits. These advantages are seen most prominently in people who have already experienced liver damage as a result of steroid use, alcoholism, improper diet, and high cholesterol.

Though research into TUDCA is still being conducted, there is plenty of evidence that indicates its potency as a liver-protecting agent. For instance, in 2010, a study from Spain published within "Cell Death and

Disease" evaluated the effects of TUDCA in patients with partial liver removals and non-steatonic livers.[53] Since it is common for both steatonic and non-steatonic livers to experience slow recovery following a partial liver removal, scientists found that TUDCA has the potential to protect the organs from regeneration failure and further injury. The effect is linked to the minimization of stress on the endoplasmic reticulum within the liver.

Another double-blind study published in 2013 in the Journal of Huazhong Science and Technology examined the efficiency of TUDCA in the treatment of scarring or fibrosis within the liver.[54] They found that the substance was more effective and safer than pharmaceutical UDCA when it came to treating cirrhosis. TUDCA is a natural supplement. It's clear that TUDCA can have a valuable part to play in protecting and repairing the liver and the surrounding lymphatic systems of the body.

TUDCA can promote good cellular function and protect the liver, reducing your chances of suffering from an impaired immune system. In other words, TUDCA could be beneficial not only for those suffering from Lyme disease but those who want to prevent chronic illness in the first place.

TUDCA can also indirectly boost the immune system, lowering your chances of falling victim to the symptoms of Lyme disease.[55]

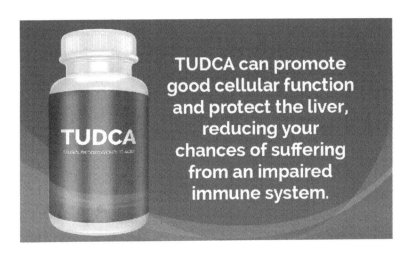

TUDCA can promote good cellular function and protect the liver, reducing your chances of suffering from an impaired immune system.

REAL CLIENTS WHO HAVE BENEFITTED FROM TUDCA:

"What do I say to someone who has completely changed my life in so many ways? I find it emotional to put down in words how grateful I am to have found you!

I am feeling better than I have in more than 8 years! I am eating smarter and healthier – which has a direct effect on my family. The 4 of us are feeling better and my Mom has changed her diet and lifestyle as well.

8 years or so ago I was slowly spiraling downhill. Strange symptoms were occurring and each and every doctor I turned to told me there was nothing wrong with me. My blood work was great and I was not overweight. I did not drink in excess and never smoked. Why was I depressed, off balance, not sleeping, imbalanced hormonally, experiencing brain

fog, ears ringing, joint and muscle pain, neck and jaw pain, and the list goes on! I was diagnosed with TMJ, Meniere's Disease, IBS, constipation, depression, anxiety, etc. Doctor's turned to pills, which made me feel worse.

Fast forward to 2015... My neighbor got a new puppy and I volunteered to take him out during the day for him. In turn, he asked if he could buy me a book written by Dr. Jay Davidson. He told me he thought Dr. Davidson could help me with what I was going through. He knew Dr. Davidson had helped his own wife and had a great book that he thought I would enjoy. I BELIEVE things are put in your life for a reason. I read this book and it was about me! I finished the book in a few short days and was on the phone making an appointment shortly after.

By listening to me on the phone and hearing all I had been through, Dr. Jay immediately knew what to test for and how to start treatment. I was on a plan that was straightforward and no one could put a price on. I was healing almost immediately and still am to this day. During each and every appointment he gave me the plan and explained in detail why we were adding or adjusting as we moved forward. I am beyond grateful for everything Dr. Jay has taught me. I cannot put into words how thankful I am for my personal journey of healing." ~Mary Kay

After working with Mary Kay, her husband Gary came to me and told me that he lost 25 pounds just by

45

following some of the protocols she was doing. He said something along the lines of: If you help me that much and I'm not working with you I can only imagine if I work with you one on one. From that point forward, I started working with Gary as well.

Gary and Mary Kay are successful realtors and Gary was a social drinker with some heart issues including arrhythmias and heart "pounding." I identified that it seemed to be the liver that was the culprit of his heart symptoms. I had been experimenting with TUDCA on some clients with surprisingly great results. One of our appointments I had him start taking one capsule of TUDCA with a meal, twice a day. On our next phone call, 30 days later, he started the conversation off, "doc, we need to talk." He continued to say that since taking the TUDCA, he was no longer able to feel his heart pounding and was worried that he couldn't feel the "beat" anymore. I explained to Gary that you are not supposed to feel your heart pounding or beating out of your chest. This client experience shows significant improvement with just less than 30 days of TUDCA. It was certainly a game changer for Gary.

Another client, Terri, who I could have put her in the "extreme case" category with my wife when we first started working together, had a lot of sensitivities. After having her start TUDCA, she informed me that she was getting massive amounts of drainage down the back of her throat, so much that it was almost making her choke. In the end, this helped clear Terri's drainage issues in ways I had not seen before. Terri's experience with TUDCA really helped me to see how opening the liver bile duct area impacted the lymphatic system and specifically the head/brain drainage! She got TUDCA for her whole family too!

Go to www.DrJayDavidson.com/FixLyme for recommended resources.

HEAT UP THE LIVER BILE DUCT!

One of my favorite things to do and recommend first thing in the morning is to take a mini infrared heating pad and strap it over my liver bile duct area (see picture below). The infrared pad that I have found to work best is sold by a company called Therasage. Therasage produces all of their products ensuring that they emit as low electromagnetic fields (EMFs) as possible, and have full spectrum infrared pads. Infrared is able to penetrate the tissues deeper than the conventional heating pad, which will usually come with high EMF risks.

The reason I love to put the pad over the front lower right ribcage is that the deep heat helps movement of the bile in the liver bile duct area. While most of us are sleeping, usually between the hours of two and four in the morning, the liver is in high detoxification mode. By heating up the liver bile duct area first thing in the morning, the movement of bile will increase and will help with phase 3 detoxification. An added benefit is that it usually helps you to poop and generally speaking, the morning is a great time to poop and "get things going".

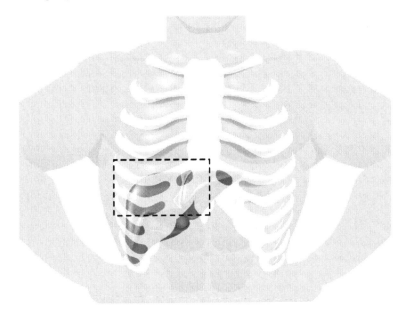

I generally will keep the infrared heating pad on my body anywhere between 30-90 minutes depending on what I'm doing on a setting of seven. I recommend starting out around a setting of four to ensure the body is handling it OK before increasing the temperature. Also, it is important to make sure to have a shirt between the pad and your skin to avoid burning your skin. I do not recommend the pad to directly contact your skin.

PHYSICAL MASSAGE OF THE LIVER AREA

Within the same areas I recommend to put the

infrared heating pad on, you can also perform a physical light trigger point massage. To do so, find the spot just below the right lower rib cage from the midline over to the side of the body (see picture below). You can do this yourself or have another person help you with it. Press down about a ½ inch or so, feeling for any hard or ropey-like areas. When you feel them, press directly on them and hold on that area for about 10-15 seconds before releasing and moving onto another area.

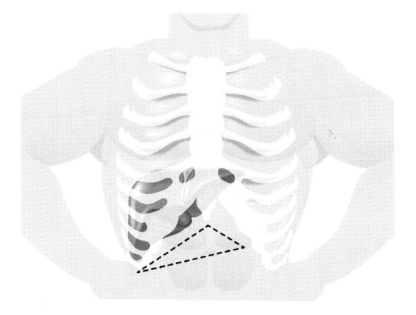

The physical massage technique was a big helper for my wife during her healing process. This is usually helpful the first couple times you do it. Once you loosen up the areas, the less you will need to do it. It is a fantastic, simple tool for anyone struggling! Don't be surprised either if you hear some gurgling while you do it as it is usually the bile duct moving bile after breaking through clogged areas.

While you are at it, you can also physically massage the colon too. Just make sure to massage it in the direction of the colon excretion! Start by lying down on your back. Again, you can massage yourself or have someone help you. Some people prefer another person help to do it because it allows them to relax their muscles and therefore receive a more effective massage. Start on the lower right side of the abdomen, near the hipbone. Gently, slowly, and somewhat firmly apply a massaging pressure into the abdomen as you move upward, about one inch above the belly button. Then, move across from right to left until you get to the other side of the abdomen. From there, start going downward until you get to the left hipbone. The pattern is in the clockwise direction that resembles an upside down "U" shape. Repeat this 3-4 times.

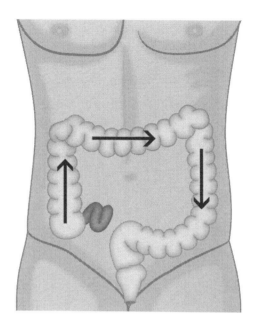

Coffee Enemas

I wrote extensively about Coffee Enemas in my first book, #1 international bestseller, *5 Steps to Restoring Health Protocol*™. I want to fill in the gaps I have seen since publishing that book and add more advancement in this area.

Frequently Asked Questions about Coffee Enemas:

What if I am not able to hold the coffee enema in for 15 minutes?

There are usually three possible reasons for this. First, you may not be putting the enema tube in far enough. If the enema tube tip is to close to the rectum/anal area (i.e. not far enough in), it will give you the feeling that you need to poop. I recommend inserting the tube into the rectum about six inches. In some cases, eight inches might work better.

The second reason you may be having a hard time holding the coffee enema is due to allowing the coffee enema solution flow too fast into the colon. Try slowly letting the liquid into the colon and as needed clamp the solution off to give your body a few seconds to gather itself. Also make sure not to put the enema bucket or bag up too high. It is typically best to keep it about two-to-three feet above not recommended to be higher.

The third reason you may not be able to hold the enema for up to 15 minutes is that you may be putting too much liquid in. I generally recommend that you make a coffee enema solution of four cups of water to four tablespoons of coffee. Then, do two coffee enemas back to back, by putting, at most, two cups of liquid in at a time. If it is challenging to hold the enema for 15 minutes, try reducing the liquid amount to anywhere between ¾ - 1 ½ cups.

What is the best coffee to use?

There are a few brands that seem to be great for coffee enemas. In my opinion, it is important to find either air roasted or lightly roasted coffee beans. I much prefer "whole" bean coffee that you grind yourself. I believe organic or at least pesticide and chemical spray free is extremely important as well. It is best to test it out, as everyone's body is not the same.

Go to www.DrJayDavidson.com/FixLyme for recommended resources.

What else can I do to help the effectiveness?

There are many herbs and supplement products that can help target the bile to soften it to get a better release. These products usually do not need to be taken immediately before the enema. These products usually work best when you are consistently taking them daily to keep the bile softer and flowing better.

TUDCA, as mentioned earlier, is a great tool. Red beetroot, choline, DPP-IV (dipeptidyl peptidase IV) enzyme, lipase enzyme, dandelion root and milk thistle are more great ingredients that help the bile duct area. Most supplement companies have a gallbladder/bile duct type formula, which may help with the effectiveness of coffee enemas.

Infrared heat is great to use before and during coffee enema. As mentioned previously, you can use an infrared heating pad in the morning over the liver bile area, around 30-60 minutes before a coffee enema. You even have the option of using it while you are laying down doing a coffee enema too.

Can you walk me through an example of how to do a coffee enema?

Let's say you wake up in the morning and you would like to have coffee enema in your routine on certain days. What I would suggest to do is to get up and make the coffee enema solution up.

- Grind up four tablespoons of whole coffee beans.
- Boil two cups of filtered water in an electric water kettle or on the stove.
- Put the freshly ground coffee in an eight cup French Press and add the boiling water. Let the mixture sit in the French Press with the cover on for 15 minutes.
- After 15 minutes, push the French Press filter down and pour the coffee into a measuring cup. You should have two cups of prepared coffee. Add filtered water until you reach four cups total. This reduces the temperature of the coffee and allows you to use it quicker.
- *Note: If you don't have a French Press, filter the coffee grounds with a fine strainer (sieve) or cheesecloth. Do not use a coffee filter because they remove the palmitates.*
- Add five-to-ten drops of tangerine essential oil to the solution. Tangerine essential oil helps to get a greater liver/bile duct release.
- Add ½ - 1 tsp. Himalayan sea salt to the solution as well. Himalayan sea salt is a great way to get minerals into the body.
- Optional: add 1 tbsp. of molasses to the solution too. Molasses helps allow the body to hold the coffee enema solution in the body longer and help to clear out more solids.

After the solution is made and cooling down, take some carbon as a binder 30 minutes before the coffee enema. Then put the infrared heating pad on at a setting of four-to-seven (not directly on skin) on your lower front right rib cage area, also 30 minutes prior. I will often leave the heating pad strapped on around my torso while I do the enema as well. Assuming the coffee solution is not too warm, proceed with your first coffee enema with about 1½ cups of liquid and attempt to hold it for 15 minutes. Gently release the coffee from your bowels on the toilet for a couple of minutes. Then, repeat with second enema of about 1½ cups of liquid and trying to hold it again for 15 minutes. Then again, gently release it on the toilet. When you are finished, take some more carbon charcoal again.

It all absorbed, but nothing really came out...what do I do now?

Occasionally your body does not release much liquid for the amount you put into the colon. That is usually a sign that the body is dehydrated and sucked the liquid up from the colon. This also more likely to happen if you do coffee enemas in the evening time as the colon is in more of an absorptive mode in the evening and is more in an expelling mode in the morning, which is why most people poop in the morning. Occasionally the colon will react and clamp down on the muscles to hold it in as well. If this happens, it is nothing to freak out about, just breath, relax and hydrate.

I feel like a wreck after the coffee enemas...why is that?

It is not the caffeine! When coffee is absorbed via the rectum from a coffee enema, it is processed much differently than coffee you intake orally. For example, caffeine you ingest while drinking coffee can be hard on your adrenal glands. The caffeine has no affect on your adrenals when it is administered rectally in an enema.

I believe that this can occur when the liver bile duct system is extremely clogged up. This also can happen when there are large amount of parasites in the bile duct area and/or high amounts of toxins. Coffee enemas are great to improve the mobility, but sometimes when things are so clogged up, it can make you feel like a wreck afterwards. You can still do coffee enemas to help open up the clogged pipes, just put half the amount of liquid in and/or put half the amount of coffee in.

If you still feel this way even after reducing the liquid and making the solution less potent, it is best to consult with a functional medicine doctor who can further assist you.

Why am I seeing funny looking things in my stool?

Coffee enemas are known to help clear out parasites. It is also possible to clear out built up sludge. It is generally difficult to see exactly what comes out of the coffee enema in the toilet, as the liquid in the toilet is coffee colored. For those who choose to dig through it or poop over top of a strainer, parasites will sometimes be in the stool after a coffee enema.

How does a coffee enema benefit me?

Coffee enemas work because the hemorrhoidal veins in the descending colon dump into the portal system via the hepatic portal vein. The coffee uses the hepatic portal vein as a direct connection to the liver. The caffeine and cholerectics present in coffee cause the liver and bile duct system to release bile into the colon and increases the flow of bile. This allows your body to use the bile created in your liver to get rid of toxins. The palmitates in the coffee are responsible for increasing glutathione, which is the body's strongest antioxidant and detoxifier. Surprisingly, coffee enemas are also one of the more effective tools to reduce pain in the body as well.

ACTIVATED CARBON

Available for purchase at most health food stores and even local pharmacies, activated carbon is most commonly used for emergency treatments. This substance offers a solution in specific cases of drug overdoses and poisonings, as it prevents substances from being absorbed further into the body. However, the more that we explore the possibilities of activated carbon, the more we see it's amazing potential. This 100% natural substance cures gastrointestinal problems, is a natural disinfectant, and can help to detoxify the body.

Taken orally, activated carbon granules are one of the finest adsorptive agents in the world. They are equipped with an incredible ability to neutralize and extract huge amounts of toxins, chemicals, and gasses.

The History of Activated Carbon

Although much of the buzz surrounding activated carbon has emerged in recent years, the substance has actually been used for centuries. One of the first recorded uses of carbon for medicinal purpose was recorded at around 1500 BC, in Egyptian papyri. Ever since then, healers across the globe have been using activated carbon to improve health and soak up poisons through a process known as "adsorption."

Physicians have used carbon for everything from epilepsy treatments to anthrax cures. When the development of activated carbon emerged in the 20th century, many medical journals began researching its properties with zeal, noting its effective antidotal effects. In fact, in 1831, Professor Touery in the French Academy of Medicine drank a lethal dose of strychnine and survived. To the amazement of his colleagues, he had combined the poison with a dose of activated carbon.

Today, activated carbon is used in hospitals and homes as an antidote for poison, a detoxifying agent, and a cure for many common ailments.

How Does Activated Carbon Work?

Activated carbon is a completely natural product that can be obtained from the carbonization of organic matter. Often, it is made by applying heat to coconut, bamboo, hardwood, olive pits, peat moss, and other natural substances. The substance begins as typical carbon (aka charcoal), before being "activated" with oxidizing gasses.

Activated carbon is a type of carbon substance that possesses a huge surface area, and a potent negative charge.[56] The negative charge of the carbon allows it to draw other substances towards the large surface area, and hold them there so that they cannot be absorbed into the body. The carbon consumed binds with chemicals whose molecules are set with positive charges and its vast system of tiny pores trap chemicals and speed up their elimination from the body. These positively charged ingredients can range all the way from pesticides to mycotoxins (such as mold) and aflatoxin B1.[57] Once the chemicals have attached themselves to the carbon, they can be passed naturally through the gastrointestinal system. Due to its incredibly porous nature, activated carbon is estimated to be able to reduce up to 60% of any poisonous substances being absorbed in the human body.

Activated carbon does not work by absorbing toxins. Instead, this substance works through the chemical process of adsorption.[58] The term "absorption" refers to the reaction of elements, including chemicals, toxins, and nutrients – that are soaked into the blood stream. On the other hand, "adsorption" is the process where elements bind with, or onto, a surface.

It is important to note that carbon can sometimes bind with good stuff too, as toxins and poisons are not the only substances that are positively charged. With that in mind, it is often a good idea to avoid taking it within an hour of additional supplements. Most experts suggest taking carbon pills alongside a sauna or exercise session. Taken properly, these supplements should absorb many of the toxins in your GI tract and gut.

Keep in mind, however, that when you consume activated carbon, you should also drink around 12-16 glasses of water per day. Activated carbon can quickly cause dehydration without adequate hydration. The more hydrated you are, the more it will help to flush away toxins quickly and prevent constipation.

Refreshing the Skin with Activated Carbon

Carbon is not only being used across the world for medical reasons as beauticians are boasting its benefits too. Externally, this adsorbent substance can easily capture and remove dirt, oil, and other micro particles that might be damaging your skin. Not only is it suitable for all skin types, but activated carbon can be used in masks, soaps, and scrubs to deep-clean and unclog pores for a more radiant appearance. Just remember that if you want to use activated carbon in your beauty routine, you should look for high-quality ingredients.

If clearer skin wasn't enough of a reason to consider using activated carbon externally, how about the fact that it's known to promote a range of other positive skin results? Activated carbon can:

- Eliminate itchiness from the skin caused by irritants or allergies
- Reduce body odor on underarms as a natural deodorant and disinfectant
- Minimize odor on feet, scalp, and even breath
- Scrub away cellulite
- Treat acne for clearer skin
- Make pores smaller
- Rid your hair of unwanted toxins, and add extra volume
- Speed the healing of wounds

To make a simple activated carbon mask, mix two capsules of carbon with just enough apple cider vinegar or filtered water to create a paste. Apply the paste to your neck and face, and leave in place for fifteen minutes before gently washing the mix away. Remember that activated carbon can be drying, so follow your routine with coconut oil to regain moisture in your skin.

Other Uses For Activated Carbon

1. Whiten Stained Teeth

If you have found your teeth becoming stained from wine, coffee, or other problematic substances over the years. Activated carbon may be the solution. This dark substance helps to promote good oral health and whiten teeth by balancing the pH balance within your mouth, helping to prevent gum disease, bad breath, and cavities. The tiny granules of activated carbon that you rub onto your teeth adsorb plaque and other microscopic substances to provide an all-natural bright smile.

Add the charcoal to a regular toothbrush and brush how you normally would. However, you might use a separate toothbrush for your carbon, as it can leave you with some stained bristles.

2. Treat Hangovers and Alcohol Poisoning

Although activated carbon cannot be used to directly adsorb alcohol, it is useful for removing other toxins from the body quickly. Alcohol is not often consumed in its purest form, which means that sweeteners and other chemicals are commonly added. Activated carbon can remove the toxins that enter the body alongside the alcohol, reducing the chance of poisoning and illness.

Studies have even shown that when activated carbon is taken in conjunction with alcohol, it can limit the alcohol concentration that is held within the blood.[59] The First Aider's Guide to Alcohol by Princeton University indicates that activated carbon should be administered in some situations pertaining to alcohol.[60] Usually, the substance is used when a patient is showing signs of acute alcohol poisoning, or is unconscious.

3. Alleviate Bloating and Gas

Activated carbon is frequently used to fight back against gastrointestinal problems and stomach discomfort. A study conducted by the American Journal of Gastroenterology discovered that activated carbon treatments can prevent the onset of intestinal gas following gas-producing meals.[61] When taking activated carbon for stomach issues, you can either take the substance in liquid, pill, or powder form.

4. Water and Air Purification

If you have ever owned a pitcher with a built in water filter, you may have noticed some of the tiny black specs of activated carbon that can escape from time to time. For the very same reasons that activated carbon is used to filter toxins from the digestive tracts of animals and humans, carbon can also filter impurities from water. Perhaps most importantly, a study from the Canadian Dental Association found that activated carbon filters for water were capable of removing some fluoride from tap water. Reducing our exposure to fluoride is essential for proper immune system functioning, as well as a healthier liver and kidneys.

Furthermore, activated carbon is also a useful solution for air filtration. The substance is odorless, easy to use, and capable of capturing a majority of airborne contaminants. My wife and I have an air filter in our bedroom with activated carbon as part of the filtration system and well as the one in my daughter's bedroom. Since EMF's are a big concern with air filters, make sure to find a brand that has low EMF's as well.

Go to www.DrJayDavidson.com/FixLyme for recommended resources.

5. Treating Stings and Bites

In the summer when stings and bites can be more common, activated carbon can be a blessing. Mixed with water or aloe, activated carbon can create a poultice, or a paste, that effectively draws the poisonous substances out of stings and insect bites.

When administered quickly, within a few minutes of the initial injury, activated carbon can reduce both swelling and pain. Of course, the nature of the injury should be monitored over time as allergic reactions and other problems can indicate the need to visit a qualified health professional. If you see excessive swelling, red streaks under the skin, or an unusual

color around the wound, consult with a doctor immediately.

6. Statin Drug Alternative

Studies conducted in labs and clinics across the globe have shown that activated carbon can be effective at reducing bad cholesterol (LDL), and increasing good cholesterol (HDL). In one particular study, the total cholesterol of volunteers decreased by 25% – with LDL (bad) cholesterol falling by 41%, and HDL (good) cholesterol increasing by 8% over four weeks.[62]

During the course of the study mentioned above, participants were required to consume three doses of eight grams of activated carbon each for the study period. As we mentioned above, however, activated carbon should not be consumed immediately following the consumption of supplements or prescription medication as it may prevent proper absorption.

7. Slow the Aging Process

Finally, though we all know that aging is a natural process that we all need to go through at some point, it is worth noting that there are some ways you can slow the hands of time. Activated carbon can be used to help prevent the common cellular damage that occurs within the liver and kidneys of an aging human being, while supporting healthy adrenal glands. Cleansing the body of the chemicals and toxins we are exposed to on a regular basis with activated carbon can effectively help us to look and feel younger.

Better Than Activated Carbon!

New breakthroughs have been made with carbon, specifically modifying the natural compounds of fulvic acid and humic acid to allow them to work systemically in the body. This means that it will not only work in the digestive tract like regular activated carbon, but will also cross into the human cell and cross the blood brain barrier.

This product has advanced functional medicine far beyond anything I have ever witnessed clinically. As much as activated carbon was a great tool for many years, it will have to take a back seat to the bioactive carbons!

These bioactive carbons not only bind onto to toxins such as heavy metals, mold, ammonia and pesticides, but they also donate carbon molecules to help support the basic backbone of life. 96% of our bodies are composed of carbon, hydrogen and oxygen. Bioactive carbons are life giving and support cellular function and repair down to the mitochondrial level.

Unlike activated carbon, bioactive carbon can be taken with or without food, as it does NOT bind onto vitamins and minerals as activated carbon does.

Go to www.DrJayDavidson.com/FixLyme for my carbon supplement recommendations.

DRAINING THE BRAIN

The brain relies on the lymphatic system, which in turn relies on the liver bile duct system. There are a couple favorites of mine that help with brain drainage. Number one is getting adequate sleep. It is important to do everything you can to protect that time and optimize it since sleep is the time when the brain drains the glymphatic fluid.

To help with brain drainage, put a drop of frankincense essential oil with a carrier oil like jojoba or fractionated coconut oil and apply to the temple, across the forehead (just on the top of the eyebrows) to the other temple. Do the same across the base of the skull (top part of the neck).

Frankincense, or boswellia, helps with brain drainage. I have seen clients with massive migraine issues get a tremendous amount of relief by using this simple technique.

The anise plant, Pimpinella anisum, and more specifically the stems, are extremely beneficial in helping to promote brain drainage quickly. This is great to pair with Desmodium molliculum, which is a perennial herb from South America.

My wife, Heather, was not able to fly on airplanes for four years due to anxiety. My wife grew up taking trips with her family and traveling to Florida every year. When we met, we traveled together for six years, then all the sudden she had this debilitating anxiety from just thinking about being on a plane, never mind actually being on a plane. She stopped flying and two years later our daughter was born, which is when the bottom fell out. In the end, the anxiety was a warning sign of what was to come and unfortunately at the time we did not dig deep to find the root cause. As my wife got better, and four years passed of no flying, her anxiety disappeared and she was able to fly again.

After being on multiple flights with no issues, we were sitting on the airplane waiting for them to close the airplanes doors to take off. We both caught a horrible cleaner type smell and Heather started to feel uncomfortable. I was holding her hand as she started to get clammy and began to fidget in her chair. I asked her if she was okay and she said she was feeling anxious. Just then, I knew it was the chemical exposure triggering the anxiety and associated symptoms.

We pulled out the Desmodium molliculum herb, as we were not yet aware of the benefits of Pimpinella anisum, and she took two doses, 15 minutes apart. She was going to take a third dose, but by then the anxiety was significantly reduced to the point of almost gone. About an hour into the flight, I had her take some activated carbon as well.

We later found out that it was the person sitting behind us that wiped down all three seats behind us with a Clorox disinfectant wipe. The toxicity exposure set my wife over the edge. I believe that there are unexpected situations you can get thrown into and it's important to be prepared. I love traveling with activated carbon and some different essentials oil as well. You never know when you are going to walk into a moldy building.

As my wife has continued to express healing and health, she is stronger now than ever and those types of situations, hardly even phase her now.

AMMONIA BUILD UP

Ammonia is an extremely alkaline toxin that can affect many different areas of the body including the brain, joints, heart, and liver. My wife never felt well with drinking alkaline water of about pH 8 to maybe pH 9. That was something that puzzled me for a while. After researching, I finally realized that she has pockets of ammonia toxin built up throughout her body. The attempt to drive the body to a more alkaline state only made the ammonia worse. Through working with other clients with Lyme and undiagnosed chronic illness, I have found ammonia build up to be a common issue.

If you are practitioner who continues to hit walls with your clients, or if you are a patient yourself and find it difficult to follow any protocol without having strange reactions, consider toxic ammonia buildup. This is why it only makes matters worse for Lyme suffers when their doctors try to force their bodies into an alkaline state. While the root of the problems are

69

usually acidic, the key is to drain the body's alkaline-ammonia areas first. This removes the buildup of the toxin and allows the body to heal.

Once you have drained the ammonia, the second step is to remove what is causing the ammonia buildup in the first place. There are two primary issues that I see causing ammonia in my clients: parasites and Lyme disease.

Go to www.DrJayDavidson.com/FixLyme for my preferred ammonia drainer.

WATER

Along with its wide range of benefits, drinking water will help the body to function optimally and assist in keeping the drainage pathways moving. Since my last book, *5 Steps to Restoring Health Protocol™*, I have been on an experimental journey the last few years in search of the "answer" for what water is best to drink, and have purchased many different filtration systems along the way.

In my last book I brought attention to the ZeroWater® gravity filtration, which I later discovered through my own experience that it would only filter about five gallons of water before needing a replacement filter! It would start having a sour taste, which I would assume the filters were starting to become bound with total dissolved solids (TDS) and chemicals.

Let's discuss the two aspects of water to consider:

chemistry and physics. Most discussion is around the chemistry of water, which is where filtration comes in. I covered this topic in my book 5 *Steps to Restoring Health Protocol*™.

The area that deserves equally as much attention is the physics of water. There have been a few researchers that have helped to pave the way in this category. Dr. Gerald Pollack, the author of the Fourth Phase of Water, discovered what he calls the "exclusion zone water" or what I would refer to as structured water. He stated that one of the properties of exclusion zone water is that it acts like a battery as it can store energy inside of it. Another pioneer in the area of physics in regards to water was Dr. Masaru Emoto.

Structured water is often referred to as hexagonal water where six water molecules are attached together in a hexagonal type shape. This can be achieved by vortexing water, using sacred geometry (some refer to as the Fibonacci numbers) and certain stones and gems.

Those that measure the chemistry side of water are usually not measuring the physics and vice versa. I believe we can find a middle ground to both sides. I like the idea of a whole house water-structuring device that is easily installed by a plumber to your water line before the water splits to hot and cold pipes. When my wife and I did this in our home, we immediately noticed that our water stopped smelling and tasting like dirt.

It's critical to understand that because water holds energy, when you filter out chemicals, which is really reducing the amount of chemicals in the water, and not 100% removing them, such as fluoride. The energy of that chemical is still in the water, a lot like how homeopathic remedies are created. Structuring your water will remove that harmful energy and frequency.

In addition to the whole house water-structuring device, you can also consider adding a water filtration device before you drink your water. Changing the chemistry of water will not remove the physics of the water. In other words, if you structure the water and than filter it, the filtration will not remove the structure of the water!

I currently recommend a whole house water-structuring device with a point of service water filtration device. You can additionally add a whole house water filtration device as well.

Go to www.DrJayDavidson.com/FixLyme to see my water recommendations.

There is very exciting research going on in regards to the topic of aquaporins. Aquaporins were discovered in 1992 as being the channels that selectively conduct water molecules in and out of the cell, while at the same time stopping the passage of ions and other solutes. The discoverer of aquaporins, Peter Agre, was awarded a Nobel prize in 2003 for his discovery. Further research in this area should demonstrate what water is able to get into and out of our cells and what factors improve or hinder this process. True hydration is when the water we ingest is getting into our cells.

LYMPHATIC MASSAGE

I believe there are two parts to ultimately restoring your health. The first is to identify and remove what the upstream causes are to your health issues in the first place. The second is use natural tools to minimize the symptoms as you are working upstream. The second one helps you to live more of a normal life versus feeling like you got hit by a train during treatment. Lymphatic massage helps significantly with the second one.

Lymphatic massage, also referred to as manual lymph drainage (or just lymphatic drainage), is typically used for lymphedema. Lymphedema can occur after trauma or surgery, such as removal of lymph nodes with breast cancer treatments. While I do not feel everyone needs to get lymphatic massages, those who are suffering from a chronic illness such as Lyme who also have swollen lymph nodes, puffy inflamed tissue, or fluid built up under skin can benefit from this.

IMPROVE YOUR CLOSENESS WITH YOUR SPOUSE

There is definitely power in human connection and especially with physical touch. If you are looking to build a closer relationship with your spouse, offering them a massage in the evening before bed can be one step in the process, which has many other benefits as well.

CHAPTER 4. SECRET #2 KILLING PARASITES

I appreciate those that are spreading the word about Lyme disease and the devastation that it can cause on someone's health and life. I see in some cases with those suffering and doctors treating Lyme that Lyme disease becomes the "only" goal and objective to kill.

I would like to be clear that I have no issues with Lyme disease treatment, and as I mentioned there is such a broad spectrum of treatments available from pharmaceutical to herbal to everything in between.

You are most likely reading this book to heal from Lyme disease or help a family member or friend heal from Lyme disease. The most important thing right now is re-establishing your health. In order for that to happen, you or the person suffering needs to identify or find a doctor or health coach to help identify the sources to your health issues and who will create a protocol that is customized to your situation.

Rarely is Lyme disease the only issue when someone is struggling with health issues. I have repeatedly seen the same issue with almost all of my clients, and the issue is something my wife struggled with as well...

Parasites! Roundworm, threadworm, tapeworm, hookworm, pinworm, liver flukes, *Blastocystis hominis, Cryptosporidium, Giardia*...you name it!

THREE MAIN CLASSES OF PARASITES:

1. Protozoa

Protozoa are single cell microscopic organisms that can be either parasitic or free-living. These creatures can multiply within humans, helping to ensure their survival, and allow for the development of serious infections. Commonly, transmission of protozoa from one human to another occurs through the fecal-oral route. For instance, if someone drinks water contaminated with fecal matter. Protozoa that live in the blood or tissue of humans or animals can be transmitted through the bite of an insect.

2. Helminths

Helminths are larger, multi-celled organisms that are often visible to the naked eye, particularly when fully grown. Similar to protozoa, helminths can be parasitic or free living, but they cannot multiply in humans within their adult form. Helminths are often separated into thorny-headed worms, flatworms, and roundworms.[63]

3. Ectoparasites

Finally, ectoparasites is a term that can be used to describe mosquitos, but is often intended to include organisms such as fleas, ticks, lice, and mites that burrow into human skin.[64] These are multi-celled organisms (often insects) can also transmit parasites through biting and stinging.

Research has shown that parasites can host bacteria (like Lyme disease) and viruses inside of them. This is extremely important to understand. If the only treatment you do is for Lyme disease and there is a parasite issue, you will hit a wall as the parasite is protecting the bacteria. Parasites can have fungus & mold spores in them replicating as well.[65]

This is can be why you are still sick from mold, especially if you were in a moldy environment such as at work or home and have parasite issues. Despite removing yourself from the moldy environment, you can still deal with mold biotoxins as the parasites can have mold spores inside of them.

It is important to note that parasites are also sponges for heavy metals. If you have had a heavy metal test performed, and it showed up low or even negative, it could be a false negative. This could be due to your body hosting parasites since they will absorb a massive amount of heavy metals. It is important to clear the build up of parasites out of the body so you can detoxify and clear the heavy metals out too.

I realized there is a modern day epidemic issue with parasites when I got two 20-inch worms out of me. I still remember that moment, being grossed out, but thankful they are not in me anymore. My mind started connecting the dots with parasites to many tough cases I worked with in the past.

I started thinking if I have them, a relatively healthy guy, who else does?

I now realize the health issues I had since I was a child were primarily from parasites:

- Bad skin issues
- Massive bags under my eyes
- Environmental allergies, food allergies, especially dairy (I used to put apple juice on my cereal growing up)
- Hyperactivity
- Wanting to take my life when I was younger
- Sensitive digestive tract
- Prone to getting sick
- Grinding my teeth
- Just not feeling right

How many people have parasite issues?

I found a press release from the CDC on May 8, 2014 titled: Parasitic Infections also occur in the United States.[66]

"Most people think parasitic diseases occur in poor and developing countries, or are infections they might pick up on a trip to a foreign country. However, parasitic infections also occur in the United States, and in *some cases affect millions of people*. Often they can go unnoticed, with few symptoms. But many times the infections cause serious illnesses, including seizures, blindness, pregnancy complications, heart failure, and even death. Anyone—regardless of race or economic status—can become infected."

Why are parasites not detected more in the United States?

"We don't find what we don't look for" ~anonymous

Parasite testing is quite inadequate at this time in America. Most labs are slammed with 20 stool samples to get through in an hour. Training of how to identify or spot 134 different species of parasites is lacking. Only 30% of parasites are visible and many are quite small. What makes it more complicated is that some parasites release an enzyme when they die that dissolves their body. So you run a stool test three-to-seven days later, chances are if there was a parasite in there, it would be gone by now.

How Do You Get Parasites?

Food is a very common way to get parasites. Raw and undercooked meat like sushi is a common cause along with improper food handling, which can often occur at restaurants and salad bars. Salad bars are notorious for having parasites in the food sitting out. The water you drink can have parasites in them, which emphasizes the need for proper filtration. I am still blow away at the amount of people that drink tap water. The air you breathe can have things such as airborne eggs, like pinworm eggs.

Do you have a cat or a dog? Have you seen where they put their mouths? I don't know if I'd kiss where that mouth has been. There is an epidemic of parasite issues in our household pets and it seems as the attention is limited to heartworm only, however, the truth is that pets can host many different parasites.

You probably would be disgusted to know what is on that shopping cart handle you touch when you go to the store! The University of Arizona in 2011 swabbed the handles of 85 carts in four states. They found that 72% of the carts had fecal matter on them and 50% of them had E. coli.[67] I live in San Diego, California right now and it is absolutely amazing the amount of people who bring their dog to the store, riding around in shopping carts.

Of course you can't forget about traveling as well, especially overseas.

Those most likely to suffer from a parasitic infection include:

- People who have a compromised immune system or chronic illness.
- People who travel to, or live within, subtropical regions.
- People who swim in rivers, ponds, or lakes where parasites are common.
- People who work in childcare.
- People who regularly work with soil.
- People who suffer from leaky gut syndrome.

Symptoms of Parasites:

- Excess boogers in nose and scab like boogers
- Anal fissures
- Loss of appetite
- Hungry all the time, bottomless pit
- Strong sugar and processed food cravings
- Anemia
- Iron deficiency
- Vitamin B6 deficiency
- Zinc deficiency
- Mood disorders
- Depression
- Anxiety
- Suicidal thinking
- Irritability
- Increase of symptoms around a full moon
- Skin issues
- Hives
- Rashes
- Eczema
- Itchy dermatitis
- Acne
- Ulcers
- Sores
- Lesions
- Itchy mouth, nose or anus
- Teeth grinder or clenching
- Wake up in the middle of the night
- Headaches

- Sore or stiff joints
- Breathing problems
- Asthma
- Persistent gut issues
- Cramps
- Bloating
- Gas
- Sexual dysfunction
- Chronic fatigue

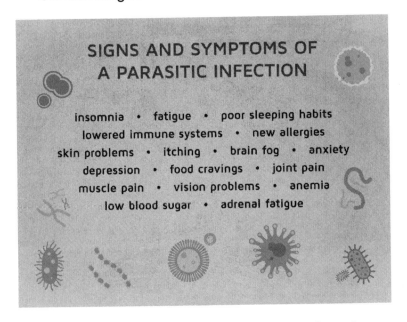

SIGNS AND SYMPTOMS OF
A PARASITIC INFECTION

insomnia • fatigue • poor sleeping habits
lowered immune systems • new allergies
skin problems • itching • brain fog • anxiety
depression • food cravings • joint pain
muscle pain • vision problems • anemia
low blood sugar • adrenal fatigue

My good friend, Dr. Todd Watts, says that if you have a pulse, you have a parasite issue. I believe it is safe to assume that if you do not do regular parasite cleanses, such as twice a year, you could develop a build up of parasites in your body.

Parasites are known to be in the digestive tract, and also throughout the body. Surprisingly enough, parasites can also be found in the liver bile duct area. These liver bile duct parasites include liver flukes, Giardia (*Giardia lamblia*), *Ascaris* (*Ascariasis lumbricoides*) and *Strongyloides* (*Strongyloides stercoralis*).[68, 69, 70]

Strongyloides is one of the causes for pyroluria, which essentially is a vitamin B6 and zinc deficiency. You can supplement with vitamin B6 and zinc to help, but until you clear the underlying parasitic infection, you will need to supplement those.

In order to open up the liver bile duct pathway, these parasites have to be addressed. An underlying parasite infestation is typically why individuals stay sensitive and clogged up.

Parasites are also a significant cause of SIBO (small intestinal bacteria overgrowth). The majority of the good bacteria in the digestive tract should be located in the large intestine (specifically the first two-thirds of the colon). Small intestinal bacterial overgrowth occurs when too much bacteria stays in the small intestine.

A popular treatment for SIBO even among some "natural" practitioners is rifaximin (aka Xifaxan®). It is touted to not harm your good bacteria as much as other antibiotics do. Clinically, I see many cases of SIFO (small intestinal fungal overgrowth) after the treatment of rifaximin, which is why I recommend steering clear of it.

COMMON SYMPTOMS DURING PARASITE CLEANSING

If you experience any of these symptoms yourself, it is important not to be alarmed. Usually, these signs are an indication of parasite die-off and that the healing process is in motion.

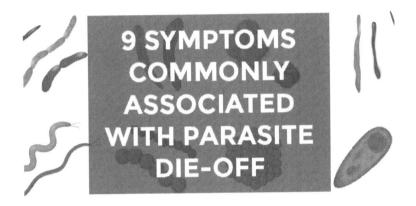

9 SYMPTOMS COMMONLY ASSOCIATED WITH PARASITE DIE-OFF

1. Crawling Sensations

It is probably not surprising to learn that a parasite cleanse is an uncomfortable experience for the parasites in your system. When worms or other sources of infection begin to realize that they are under attack, they may start to move around.

2. Headaches

Headaches are generally a brain drainage issue, but headaches can also be a result of parasites moving around inside the head.[71] In these circumstances,

84

pain may be located behind or inside of the eyes, around the ears, or all over the body.

3. Fatigue and Weakness

When you consider the fact that parasites like Giardiasis can be responsible for causing chronic fatigue syndrome, it is easier to accept that you might feel some fatigue temporarily during the process of eliminating parasites from your system.[72] It is worth noting that it takes a great deal of energy for your body to rid itself from parasites.

4. Skin Sores

Skin sores are yet another common symptom of parasite die-off. These sores can occur when the body tries to eliminate toxins at a quicker pace than is typically possible. The skin is one of the organs that can rid the body of toxins, and if too many toxins attempt to leave the skin at once, this can lead to breakages and sores. Toxins that leave the body by breaking through the skin might include eggs, parasite waste, or the parasites themselves.

5. Digestive Problems

This symptom is the most common one. Three weeks into a parasite cleanse, my stomach starting rolling and I just did not feel good. I had just arrived at a hotel to attend a conference. I was not speaking, so I had no reason to be nervous or anxious, which is what it felt like. I developed some loose stools and the next day I passed two 20-inch worms. As soon as they passed, I felt great again.

Digestive problems are issues that can start to arise when the parasite is still living within your body, but in some cases, these issues may appear to get worse when you begin your parasite cleanse. Depending on the severity of the parasite you are trying to remove, you could experience instances of bloating and diarrhea as your body attempts to eliminate all dangerous substances within. Some people may even feel strange knots or lumps in their abdomen.

6. Emotional Instability

I have had multiple clients reach out to me during parasite cleansing to let me know that they feel emotionally instable. While this may be a scary side effect, it is important to remember that it will pass once the parasites have been removed properly.

7. Easy or more Frequent Bruising

As mentioned above, when the parasites in your system feel threatened, they will start to become more restless. The result of this restlessness means that you will begin to feel the creatures moving around inside of your body, potentially looking for a new place to live. Whatever the reason for the movement inside of your body, when parasites move too close to the skin, the result can be easier bruising. You might find yourself covered in marks though you have not had any reason to bruise.

8. Cravings

Parasites feed on specific foods within your body more avidly than others. It is common to feel cravings during the first few days of cleansing. Make sure to remember it is the worms causing these cravings.

9. Respiratory Effects

Finally, the destruction of parasites in your body may cause your body to take drastic measures to remove the foreign invaders as quickly as possible. Since increasing the flow of mucous is often seen as an effective way to rid the body of other contaminants, the chances are that you will experience several respiratory symptoms like those of the common cold, including sneezing, coughing, and a runny or stuffy nose.[73]

Favorite Parasite Tools

When I got the two 20-inch worms out of me, I was using mimosa pudica seed. Mimosa pudica herb is great to help with rope worm, roundworm, biofilm, mucoid plaque, and other intestinal nematodes. The key is to get the seed form. The mimosa pudica plant is not even close to as effective as the seed form. Do not waste your money on the plant form.

Clove, neem and vidanga are extremely helpful as well with parasites. Vidanga is an herb that deserves a lot more attention and credit. It has been used in ayurvedic medicine to treat parasites for years. I am personally not a big fan of anti-parasitic drugs.

An important concept to understand with parasite cleansing is the idea of rotating formulas and not taking the same thing by itself. For instance, take some anti-parasitic herbs for a month and then change it up, at least a little. Mimosa pudica seed is an exception to this as it is a great parasite binder. I have had clients that are so riddled with worms that they will take it for a year and still see things come out.

Go to www.DrJayDavidson.com/FixLyme to see my parasite formula recommendations.

CHAPTER 5. SECRET #3 REMOVING TOXINS

MAN MADE EMR

EMR otherwise known as electromagnetic radiation is a form of energy that can cause disease and hinder healing. EMR is often mentioned as EMFs (aka electromagnetic fields), but the more accurate term is EMR. I consider EMR to be a digital source of toxicity to the body.

As the world continues to industrialize, and technological revolutions continue, there has been a huge increase in the amount of sources emitting electromagnetic radiation. Though for some people it seems that devices such as computers and cell phones make our lives easier, they also physically stress our bodies out. Anything with an EMR emission can harm your health.

For years, people have reported various health problems that have been linked back to EMR exposure. While some people report milder symptoms, and attempt to avoid the digital toxicity stress, others are severely affected. Some are affected so significantly that they can no longer live a normal life.

The World Health Organization tells us that EMR is everywhere. These energy fields negatively impact our bodies, by interfering with our own highly sensitive electrical systems. People react to EMR in different ways. Some may not notice any symptoms, while others experience a range of symptoms, including:

- Infertility, miscarriages and sexual changes
- Problems with the digestive system
- Symptoms throughout the ear nose and throat
- Depression and inability to focus
- Eye blurriness and burning
- Skin symptoms like rashes, prickling, and burning
- Limb and muscle aches
- Nervous system issues leading to sleep problems and fatigue

EMR exposure has even been linked to cancer.[74] It is also important to note that EMR exposure can also have negative effects on those suffering from chronic illness such as Lyme disease.

How EMR Interfere with Chronic Illness

Over the last couple of decades, there has been a significant rise in chronic infection and autoimmune diseases. WHO recognizes chronic disease as the major cause of disability and death around the world.

Some experts have noticed a link between the rise in EMR exposure and the growth of chronic illness. This is particularly relevant in Lyme disease, where widespread inflammation and depleted immunity interact.

If you suffer from a chronic condition like Lyme disease, you might be eating healthy, reducing stress, and maybe even taking supplements. However, you might not be thinking about the impact of the harmful products all around you. Everything you do, and everything around you, can impact your disease.

Dr. Dietrich Klinghardt found that EMR shielding was more successful at treating Lyme than any antibiotics he had tried. According to Klinghardt, EMR could be responsible for driving virulence in the microbes naturally in our bodies. In other words, electromagnetic radiation could be making internal microbes more aggressive.

Research had already shown radiation causes immunosuppression and inflammation.[75] In the body, inflammation begins with allergies, and can progress to autoimmunity. As the immune system fires at the wrong targets, it is unable to protect against a growing infection – like Lyme.

Radiation also causes myelosuppression.[76] This is the reduced output of blood cells from bone marrow, including white blood cells. White blood cells are designed for immunity. A low white blood cell count can make it harder to protect against chronic illness.

EMR, just like any toxin, can accumulate within the body. Through chronic exposure, the build up of EMR combined with an already weakened immune system such as in chronic illness can make it difficult for the body to fight infection.

EMR and the Immune System

Dr. Klinghardt believes that seven minutes of phone radiation can be enough to activate dormant Epstein Barr virus. In sufferers of chronic Lyme, there is a naturally lowered immune system.[77] Since a depressed immune system struggles to produce antibodies, it is often very difficult to fight against infection. In addition to reducing white blood cells, radiation can cause shrinkage in the thymus gland.[78] The thymus gland is responsible for the immune system, maturing white blood cells.

Radiation can also lead to the reduction of red blood cells.[79] This means that patients begin to suffer from reduced platelets, which are the substances required for clotting. On top of that, a lack of red blood cells can also lead to iron deficiency.

In cases of severe acute radiation poisoning, patients can bleed from various orifices, however, in cases of EMR exposure it is more likely that patients might suffer from easy bruising. Iron needs to be bound to red blood cells to move around the body. If iron is not bound, it provides a food source for infections. Infecting microbes can use iron for survival. This is why it is worth considering supplementing during infections. Iron deficiency, or anemia, is found in a large number of Lyme patients.

EMR and Lyme Disease

One of the most important issues to address with chronic Lyme, is exposure to electromagnetic radiation.

Most people today are engulfed in a constant bubble of dangerous EMR generated by Wi-Fi, Bluetooth devices, electricity, cell phones, and more. This EMR comes from environments all around us, every day. It stresses the immune system, and inhibits the treatment for chronic Lyme. It also breaks up DNA strands, creates stress hormones, and weakens the blood/brain barrier.[80] EMR can disrupt the way your cells function, and clog detoxification pathways in the body.

An increase in electricity in homes has created a host of new health problems that have remained unknown until recently. Studies show that electromagnetic pollution exacerbates, and even causes a range of problems.[81] EMR can contribute to disorders like autism, and cancer. They also have links with insomnia, chronic fatigue, and more.

Back in 2013, a study was published showing that EMR has a non-thermal chemical impact on human biology.[82] It damages proper biological function by pushing calcium out of our cells. EMR also damages potassium ions, which regulate brain function, and lithium, which regulates mental stability.

The permeability of the cell membranes over our

nerves, skin, and organs are affected. The intricate DNA of chromosomes have been shown to be affected by EMR too.[83] Throughout the entire human body, it seems that every biochemical process involves the precisely choreographed behavior of various EMR-sensitive atoms and molecules.

Electromagnetic Sensitivity

With over 25 years of intensive study into EMR, the Swedish government has learned a lot about EMR. Their research into electromagnetic fields has even prompted them to create a health and safety limit for exposure. This Swedish limit is set at 2.5 Mg for ELF fields, and 0.25 for VLF fields.

At this point in time, the United States government has not published any standards around EMR and electromagnetic problems. The Swedish standard is one that has been accepted around the world. This means that if you are constantly exposed to more EMR than the standard limit, you could be at risk of several health problems. While sometimes those health problems may be minimal, both acute and chronic exposure can lead to major health issues for some. The severity of your reaction, and how EMR impact your chronic illness could be connected to a specific sensitivity.

Most people who are ill with a chronic disease will notice that they are more sensitive to EMR. People with chronic illnesses like chronic Lyme disease will likely suffer more from exposure to EMR because the body is already in a dysfunctional state. The system is in turmoil, and those invisible waves add extra stress.

Electromagnetic sensitivity is often characterized by many unspecific symptoms. Those symptoms are typically attributed to exposure to a large amount of electric waves.

According to WHO, there have been a number of estimations regarding the prevalence of electromagnetic hypersensitivity (EHS) around the world. A survey across occupational medical centers suggested that only a few individuals have this problem. However, surveys of self-help groups yielded far higher results. Around 10% of reported cases of EHS have been deemed severe.[84]

The most common symptomatic reaction for someone with electromagnetic sensitivity is dermatological. Usually, a person will experience a warm, or burning sensation in the affected area. For some people, this area will be one side of the head or face. For other people, there may be a general burning throughout the entire body. Often, patients describe the sensation as similar to being sunburnt.

There are also physical signs that can appear as a result of electromagnetic sensitivity. For instance, you might suffer from blemishes, eye problems, or have especially dry skin. Below is a list of some of the symptoms commonly attributed to electromagnetic sensitivity:

- Burning or warm sensations in the face (similar to being sunburnt)
- Tingling or prickling sensations across the body or face
- Extreme dryness in the skin and mucus membranes, this might include dry eyes, throat, and mouth
- Swelling in the mucus membranes around the nose, ears, throat, and sinuses without any obvious infection
- Issues with memory-loss, concentration problems, and dizziness
- Feelings of impending cold or flu symptoms that never quite arrive
- Nausea and headaches
- Pains throughout the teeth and jaw
- Pains and aches throughout joints and muscles
- Palpitations in the heart or chest

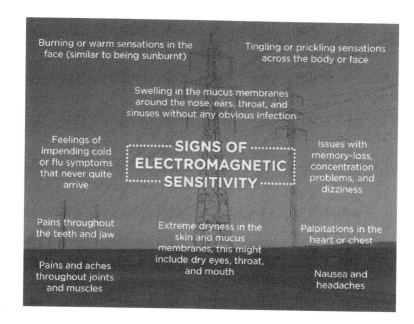

Burning or warm sensations in the face (similar to being sunburnt)

Tingling or prickling sensations across the body or face

Swelling in the mucus membranes around the nose, ears, throat, and sinuses without any obvious infection

Feelings of impending cold or flu symptoms that never quite arrive

SIGNS OF ELECTROMAGNETIC SENSITIVITY

Issues with memory-loss, concentration problems, and dizziness

Pains throughout the teeth and jaw

Extreme dryness in the skin and mucus membranes, this might include dry eyes, throat, and mouth

Palpitations in the heart or chest

Pains and aches throughout joints and muscles

Nausea and headaches

WHAT CAN YOU DO ABOUT EMR EXPOSURE?

Ultimately, most experts suggest that the link between EMR and chronic disease is significant. That means that if you want to overcome a case of chronic Lyme, your first step will be to limit your exposure to EMR as much as possible.

With so many different sources of EMR in the world today, it can be very difficult to lower your dose to nothing. However, just because you can't avoid EMR entirely, does not mean you are unable to reduce your exposure.

If you are living within a city or suburb, the chances are that you are exposed to many different EMR sources each day. Both indoors, and outdoors, you are exposed to electrical signals. If you have a lot of wireless devices in your home, it could be helpful to switch to wired technology. Corded solutions emit lower amounts of EMR, and help you to reduce your exposure. Although it often feels more convenient to buy wireless equipment, the dangers can be significant.

Other ways to reduce EMR exposure include:

44% of people sleep with their cellphone, and this leads to constant exposure to EMR during the night if it's not in airplane mode.[85] If you sleep with your phone by you, make sure to put it in airplane mode. If you don't put it in airplane mode keep your cell phone as far away from you as possible. Important note: do not charge your cell phone by you while you sleep. EMR rises significantly in the area of the phone when it's being charged.

Do not put your cell phone directly to your head/ear while speaking on it. I recommend to use speakerphone or a wired headset with a ferrite bead on it. Ferrite beads or ferrite chokes are simple hollow cylinder shaped plastic pieces with ferrite material inside that you snap onto the cord. I recommend to loop the cord through the ferrite bead twice and have it about two thirds away from the phone on the cord or one third away from the ear piece on the cord. They help to reduce the headset cord from transmitting EMR directly to your head.

Do not allow your children to use cellphones. Younger people are typically more prone to EMR problems. The brain of a child is less developed and protected than that of an adult. Their skulls are thinner, meaning that EMR penetration is easier.

Stop using of anything wireless that utilizes Bluetooth or WI-FI. I recommend using corded internet and shutting the WI-FI part off on your router, computer, tablet and cell phone. Other devices to check are speaker systems, TV's, appliances, home thermostat, security system, etc. Ask yourself how can you get rid of certain devices from your home if they are transmitting Bluetooth or WI-FI if you can't disable the Bluetooth or WI-FI. I am absolutely terrified by the idea of a smart home where everything is wireless!

Understand EMR sensitivity: Ask the people around you to limit their use of EMR devices when possible. Explain that you are sensitive to electromagnetic frequencies, and their use of certain devices could damage your recovery. The people who care about you should be willing to change their habits to help you recover faster.

Don't carry your cellphone in your pocket unless it's on airplane mode. Sometimes, you can reduce your exposure to EMR waves simply by changing habits. Keep your cellphone in a bag or purse when you're moving around. This will create some distance between the device and your body. Remember, cellphones emit EMR even when you're not using them to text or make calls.

Avoid using extension cords inside your home. Unshielded extension cords transmit EMR wherever the cord is. If you need to use extension cords and surge protectors, make sure to get shielded versions which will limit EMR.

Remove cordless phones from the house.

Avoid using LED decorative light and rope lights. The conversion of AC to DC current creates EMR. If you have solar panels, shield the conversion box or move the conversion box to an area where no one is.

Get your smart meters removed. In San Diego where I live, it was $75 to switch our electrical meter back to the traditional meter and an extra $10 a month to not have a smart meter. Way worth the investment as it was on the wall where my daughter sleeps at night.

What do I do when I am on the computer and phone most days with clients? I have my computer WI-FI and Bluetooth off. Our entire internet is wired. I avoid using my cell phone for calls as much as possible. I use Google voice aka www.hangouts.google.com to make phone calls from my computer with my wired headset.

With increasing use of technology, we are also constantly learning about the dangers of exposure to electromagnetic radiation. For now, it is safe to say that whether you are suffering from a chronic illness or not, you should limit your exposure to these dangerous waves as much as possible.

KOMBUCHA AND ELECTROMAGNETIC RADIATION

A study published within the journal of Applied Sciences and Radiation research during 2014, looked at the impact of kombucha on the trace elements in the organs of rates exposed to EMR.[86]

Within the research, there were four groups of rats. The first group was a control group exposed to no electromagnetic radiation. The second group included rates exposed to a 950hz electromagnetic radiation. That EMR was taken from a commercially available cellphone at the time. The third group included rats that were fed kombucha and not exposed to EMR. Finally, the fourth group were rats that were given kombucha, and were exposed to the same EMR as mentioned above.

In this particular study, the researchers instantly found that the rats exposed to the EMR had significantly changed levels of zinc, copper, and iron in their systems. These metals are all associated with oxidative stress management. Previous studies have indicated that EMR promotes oxidative stress, which is damaging to the entire body.

The study showed a 50% increase in iron levels within the intestines of rats exposed to EMR. At the same time, they had a 33% lower amount of zinc, and a

23% higher amount of copper. In other words, the changes weren't just small. Interestingly, the kombucha fed to the rats seemed to reduce these effects.

For the rats who had been fed kombucha and exposed to EMR, though the effects weren't completely diminished, the levels were shifted closer to those of the control group. The study also looked at the impact that EMR had on the spleen and brain, with similar results.

In their comments on the study, the authors found that the kombucha cultures the rats consumed contained two symbiotic microbes: yeasts, and xylinum. They believed that because xylinum creates cellulose from ethanol produced by yeast, that created a solution that lead to an efficient adsorbing agent. The resulting agent could adhere to metallic irons and facilitate their removal more easily.

Copper, Zinc, and Iron might not seem very important to your body on the surface, however, the way that these metals interact with each other can easily wreak havoc on your health. The study mentioned above indicates that there is now compelling evidence for people to drink more kombucha. If you are exposed to EMR regularly, or have altered zinc, copper, or iron levels, then kombucha could be the cure.

The Other Health Benefits of Kombucha

Of course, it is worth noting that kombucha has a lot

of positive benefits beyond its EMR-fighting abilities. Scientists believed that kombucha could assist with detoxification, anti-oxidation, energy production, and immunity development.[87]

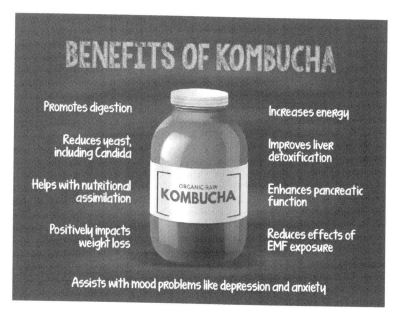

BENEFITS OF KOMBUCHA

Promotes digestion

Reduces yeast, including Candida

Helps with nutritional assimilation

Positively impacts weight loss

ORGANIC RAW
KOMBUCHA

Increases energy

Improves liver detoxification

Enhances pancreatic function

Reduces effects of EMF exposure

Assists with mood problems like depression and anxiety

MOLD TOXICITY

If any of your testing results have shown *Chlamydia pneumoniae* or mycoplasma, consider mold, as these are both typically associated with mold toxicity. Let's be very clear, it is not a mold allergy! It is a mold toxicity that causes the body to react. Technically mold is a biotoxin, which is in the same category as Lyme disease.

TOXIC MOLD EXPOSURE AND LYME DISEASE

Many people who suffer with chronic Lyme disease continue experiencing symptoms because something, often times multiple issues, are standing in the way of their recovery. If you have been treated for Lyme, but are still unwell, one of the underlying issues could be toxic mold exposure.

If you live, or work in a water-damaged area, then your body could be building up mold toxins. These toxins, known as "mycotoxins", can trigger inflammation and damage your immune system.[88] This means that exposure to mycotoxins is harmful on its own, but it can be particularly detrimental in people suffering from chronic Lyme.

According to Dr. Raj Patel, almost half of all unresolved Lyme cases could be linked to mold illness.[89] Since both conditions cause similar symptoms, like joint pain and brain fog, it can be difficult to distinguish between the two.

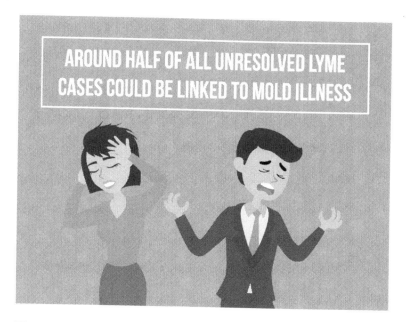

AROUND HALF OF ALL UNRESOLVED LYME CASES COULD BE LINKED TO MOLD ILLNESS

Toxic mold illness comes from exposure to water-damaged buildings. Many professionals consider "biotoxin illness", or mold illness to be a co-condition of Lyme. When the body is exposed to mold mycotoxins during a Lyme infection, the system can weaken and suffer significantly. Until recently, the Lyme medical community has not recognized the connection between mold toxicity and Lyme disease.

IDENTIFYING MOLD ILLNESS AND LYME DISEASE

Mold toxicity is a term that describes how different molds can damage humans in excess quantities. Mold is a fungi or mildew that develops when in the presence of the right environment. The chances are you have likely seen mold on anything from old food to bathroom grout and basement wood. Today, there are more than 150,000 types of mold, though not all species are harmful to humans.[90]

Mold biotoxin illness is often times referred to as Chronic Inflammatory Response Syndrome (CIRS). The reason you get ill from mold is that you inhale the spores, which reproduce within your lungs and damage your immune system. The different types of molds that are toxic to humans, and sometimes linked with Lyme disease, include:

- Stachybotrys: The most serious form of mold toxicity. This type of mold includes black mold, and can be responsible for eye irritation, respiratory issues, and central nervous system malfunction. In severe cases, black mold has been linked to nerve and brain damage, as well as cancer, and even death.[91]
- Memnoniella: Mycotoxins found alongside black mold. This substance affects both humans and animals.[92]
- *Penicillium*: A type of mold that can be found in food, dust, and decaying materials. There are over 160 species of *Penicillium*, and symptoms of exposure can include rashes, vomiting, and hair thinning.[93]
- Cladosporium: A dark-green or black substance found indoors and outdoors. There are more than 30 species of this mold. These substances cause asthma, nail fungus, and sinusitis.[94]

- Fusarium: Found in water-damaged environments. These molds are associated with infections and eye irritation. They can also cause internal bleeding, diarrhea, and reproductive issues in females.
- Mucor: Found in animal droppings and soil. The most common symptom of exposure to this mold is a lung infection.[95]
- Anternaria: Found in plants and soil. When inhaled, this mold causes allergic reactions, hay fever, and asthma.

MOLD AND MYCOTOXINS

Mold can produce substances that may be harmful to our health. Fungi produce active biological compounds that can be volatile. When these substances are released into the air, they can be inhaled, leading to serious respiratory reactions.

The most significant dangers of Mold come from poisonous elements called "mycotoxins". Over 200 different mycotoxins have been discovered in connection with common molds. There is some increasing evidence that these substances can cause DNA damage.

Some of the mycotoxins that have seen the most attention over the years are those produced by Aspergillus veriscolor and Stachybotyrs chartarum. Even in tiny quantities, mycotoxins are easily absorbed by the body. Some are so toxic that they were studied as biological warfare agents in the 1940s.

Even if the spores you are exposed to are not able to reproduce, they can still damage your health. In other words, dead spores are just as dangerous as the live ones. Scientists believe that mycotoxins help mold organisms to remain competitive in the biological environment. They kill other organisms that attempt to thrive in the same environment.

When a patient compromised by Lyme, or chronic Lyme is exposed to mycotoxins, the mold symptoms that occur can neutralize the healing solution prescribed. Your treatment plan for Lyme might be more effective if you tackle mycotoxins too.

If the reason for your continued Lyme illness is mold illness, then your home or workplace needs to be cleaned immediately. The same rules apply for anyone exposed to tick-borne illnesses. Certified mold inspectors need to be used, with state-of-the-art technology to seek out hidden sources of moisture that might trigger mold growth.

Mold Illness and CIRS

Up until recently, the connection between mold and human health has been largely ignored. Not only has the medical community failed to consider the problem that mold could be having on Lyme patients, but the impact that mold can have in general has been widely overlooked.

Today, what many experts refer to as "mold illness" may be a more complicated syndrome. This syndrome is a multi-faceted illness called "Chronic Inflammatory Response Syndrome", or CIRS. The illness "CIRS" was first identified by Dr. Ritchie Shoemaker.

During the 1990s, Dr. Shoemaker found a connection between an illness his patients had, and toxic exposure to something called Pfiesteria. Since that time, Shoemaker has linked various illnesses to toxins, organisms, and chemicals. These agents, known as "biotoxins", are often found in water-damaged buildings, and can include:

- Fungi
- Mold
- Bacteria
- Actinomycetes
- Mycobacteria
- Mold
- Mold spores
- Beta-glucans
- Endotoxins
- mVOCS (Microbial volatile organic compounds – released by micro-organisms when an adequate food supply is available).

When exposed to high enough levels of these

biotoxins, almost anyone could become ill. However, most people will recover automatically when the substance causing the problem is removed. The natural system for detoxification in our bodies, the immune system, recognizes biotoxins. Once your immune system has identified that biotoxins are causing inflammatory responses, it can begin to eliminate them.

However, some people have the "human leukocyte antigen", or HLA gene, that prevents the body from eliminating biotoxins. In these cases, the toxins remain in the body and cause a chronic response, leading to the development of CIRS. According to research from Dr. Shoemaker, around 25% of the population may develop CIRS. The only two conditions that are needed to promote this condition are:

1. Exposure to a sufficient level of biotoxins.
2. Exposure to an inflammatory event: such as Lyme disease, which causes a severe upper respiratory tract infection.

According to a report published by the Federal Facilities Council, 43% of the buildings they examined had current water damage, while 85% had previous water damage. The combination of a growing susceptibility to CIRS, and a range of water-damaged building could cause serious problems.[96]

Typically, CIRS patients experience a wide range of vague symptoms, including but not limited to:

- Chronic weakness and fatigue
- Post-exertional malaise
- Confusion and general feelings of disorientation
- Problems with memory management
- Difficulty with concentration and cognitive function
- Progressive headaches
- Lightheadedness and vertigo
- Aching in the muscles
- Cramps
- Joint pains without inflammatory arthritis symptoms
- Asthma-like illnesses which include coughing and sinus congestion
- Significant sensitivity to bright lights, blurred vision and eye tearing
- Abdominal problems such as cramping, diarrhea, and nausea
- Static shocks

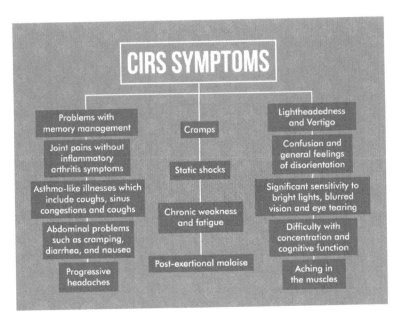

CIRS SYMPTOMS

- Problems with memory management
- Joint pains without inflammatory arthritis symptoms
- Asthma-like illnesses which include coughs, sinus congestions and coughs
- Abdominal problems such as cramping, diarrhea, and nausea
- Progressive headaches
- Cramps
- Static shocks
- Chronic weakness and fatigue
- Post-exertional malaise
- Lightheadedness and Vertigo
- Confusion and general feelings of disorientation
- Significant sensitivity to bright lights, blurred vision and eye tearing
- Difficulty with concentration and cognitive function
- Aching in the muscles

Obviously, many of the symptoms associated with CIRS are non-specific. This means it would be difficult for healthcare professionals to use them to single-handedly define the illness.

HOW TO TREAT TOXIC MOLD ILLNESS

The first step in treating toxic mold illness is to remove yourself from the contaminated environment. This either means leaving the infested place until it has been fully cleaned, or taking steps to minimize biotoxins in your home or office.

Some of the ways that you can minimize biotoxins in your current environment include:

- Fixing plumbing leaks or moisture problems as soon as possible

- Discard any absorbent materials, including carpet and ceiling tiles
- Do not paint or caulk surfaces that are contaminated with mold
- Repair and clean guttering regularly
- Keep air condition pans clean, and drain lines unobstructed
- Try to ensure that the ground slopes away from your building foundation, to reduce the risk of gathering water
- Maintain indoor humidity at between 30 and 50 percent. Venting bathrooms, dryers, and moisture-generating devices outdoors can help; use exhaust fans when you cook, clean, and even wash dishes
- Do not install carpets in any areas with perpetual moisture problems

While improving the air quality of your building, and removing potential biotoxins, it could be worth your while to introduce air sanitizers. For instance, a HEPA filter can help to remove ultra-fine particles from the air such as VOCs, mold, dust, and pet dander. Be cautious of buying air filters as many of them have extremely high EMR.

My wife and I currently have an air filter in our bedroom as well as our daughter's bedroom. We also have an air purifier in our house. An air filter is a device that pulls air into it and an air purifier is a device that puts molecules out into the air. I recommend staying away from any type of device that produces ozone. Ozone machines produce extremely high amounts of EMR and ozone is dangerous to breath in. Also ozone produces a dangerous byproduct once combined with mold spores. I much prefer a hydrogen ion air purifier. Hydrogen ions not only take care of mold spores in the air, but also help to reduce VOCs and other air toxins.

Go to www.DrJayDavidson.com/FixLyme for air filter and air purifier recommendations.

Dr. Shoemaker likes to use cholestyramine and welchol to bind internal mycotoxins. I do not agree with this approach. I have found clinically that carbon, especially bioactive carbon, works wonders for binding mycotoxins in the body.

It is important to remember that when you are using binders, you need to take steps to ensure that you maintain proper bowel function and avoid constipation. A few ways to limit your risk of constipation might include using vitamin C, and/or magnesium.

Go to www.DrJayDavidson.com/FixLyme for the best bowel movers.

Some foods even contain their own mycotoxins, which could lead to additional overgrowth in your system when you are battling against mold illness. Some foods to avoid include peanuts, corn, barley, rye, wheat, and cheese. You should also stay away from alcohol, oats, pistachios, dried fruit, cocoa, coffee, bread, sunflower seeds and beans.

Some of the most common symptoms of mold toxicity include:

- Weight gain – Some people experience weight loss, but most suffer from rapid weight gain that doesn't stop until they receive treatment.
- Brain fog, lack of concentration or cognitive function, and memory loss. Children have been found to experience drops in IQ after frequent mold exposure.[97]
- Damage to the brain caused by mycotoxins irritating the amygdala
- Nose and eye irritation (itching, redness, soreness, and bleeding)
- Dermatitis
- Asthma or respiratory infections that may lead to issues such as coughing up blood
- Fatigue, dizziness, and flu-like symptoms
- Headaches
- Vomiting and diarrhea
- Liver damage
- Damage to the immune system

While the above symptoms have been seen in people who were exposed to toxic mold spores, other symptoms may also exist. Some reports of animals that have been exposed to mold in laboratory conditions have shown other symptoms such as:[98]

- Neurotoxicity
- Reproductive cycle disruption
- Infertility
- Kidney damage

STEP 1: DISCOVERING WHERE THE MOLD COMES FROM

When it comes to removing mold from your home, the first step is to find out why the mold has accumulated in the first place. Usually, the answer will be connected to leaking, humidity over 50%, or water damage. In most homes, leaking windows or pipes, leaking roofs, and indoor flooding can explain the presence of mold. To grow, the spores need the following conditions:

- Darkness
- Warmth
- Food (cotton, drywall, wood)
- Existing spores
- Oxygen
- Time
- Moisture

Since all of the other conditions on the above list are almost always present in homes, moisture is the key cause of growth. Of course, not all mold may be as damaging to your health. The most dangerous, or toxic spores are those that produce mycotoxins,

116

substances that are responsible for causing adverse health reactions.[99]

STEP 2: FIX THE CAUSE, NOT THE SYMPTOMS

When most homeowners notice the presence of mold, they turn directly to bleach to solve the problem. However, the truth is that bleaching a surface is perhaps one of the worst things you can do in the fight against toxic mold. Though this product will clean the surface, the water in the bleach will feed the mold you can't see. Instead, you should be looking to purchase a product known as "Concrobium".

The Occupational Safety and Health Administration (OSHA), were one of the first agencies to stop recommending the use of bleach for dealing with mold problems.[100] Since then, the Environmental Protection Agency (EPA) have updated their guide to remove their once-suggested use of bleach as a means of killing spores.[101]

While bleach can kill some mold, it only works at removing the spores on the surface of your walls, tiles, or floors. However, the problem is that to ensure survival, mold spreads its roots (or Mycelia) deep into porous surfaces where the substances in bleach that kill spores cannot reach. This means that mold remediation requires a cleaner that reaches deep down into porous materials to remove the roots of the mold. At the same time, bleach contains about 90% water, a substance that mold loves. When bleach is applied to a surface, the chlorine quickly evaporates and leaves behind water, which soaks into the porous surface and feeds the mold. In other words, using bleach actually feeds the internal mold spores.

Facts to Remember about Bleach and Mold:

- In some cases, bleach can encourage toxic mold to grow further and faster due to excess moisture.
- Bleach only removes the color from mold. The surface appears clean but roots continue to grow.
- The EPA and OSHA have specifically advised against using bleach for mold remediation.
- Chlorine bleach, the bleach most commonly used in cleaning mold, is extremely harmful to surfaces. If bleach is used in a substance such as wood, it starts to weaken down the material by breaking the fibers, creating problems with the structural integrity of a home.

MOLD STORY

I believe so many breakthroughs come when my team and I work with tough cases. When you can figure out how to get the toughest of tough cases well, everyone doing better than that can get well easier. I learned this lesson from my wife originally and continue to see this as my team and I work with clients.

One specific client of mine had many sensitivities. The steps that I normally take were helping but she was not able to move beyond the sensitivities. She had a tough time with cleansing parasites as well as a tough time detoxing heavy metals even though she was very diligent. She followed instructions, had a great mindset, and yet seemed to be progressing much slower than I would have expected.

Dr. Nick, one of the brilliant doctors on our team, started working with her adult daughter and we saw similar issues with her as well. My first thought was wondering if there might be a genetic component to all of this. As time went on, I kept getting this feeling that we were missing something. She had her house evaluated for EMR (EMFs). Although in the beginning we thought mold was not an issue, I decided to revisit the topic with her. She told me that she worked from home and I asked if her daughter was ever over at her house. She said she was over a lot as they worked together. BINGO, we had a match beyond genetics: Her home! She hired a mold inspector and found aspergillis and stachybotris in her home!

The lesson here is to always be sure to consider mold. Just remember, mold can develop anytime, so even if it's been ruled out once, it could have developed after the testing was completed.

HEAVY METAL TOXICITY

Mercury, lead, cadmium, aluminum and arsenic are some of the more common heavy metals which impact us. For more information on heavy metal toxicity, see my previous book *5 Steps to Restoring*

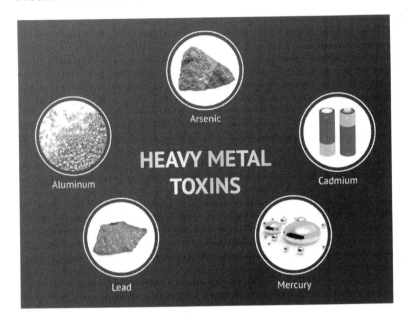

Since writing that book, I now see how much heavy metals, parasites, Lyme and mold are all related and connected. I believe the heavy metal toxicity epidemic has created a parasite epidemic. Parasites are sponges for heavy metals, which means if the body has a heavy metal toxicity issue, parasites are likely to stick around. The immune system is weakened to pathogens, but also will allow more parasites to be present in the body to deal with the heavy metal load. Remember, this is a reason heavy metal testing can be inaccurate when there are parasites presents. Parasites hide the metals in them.

DIET

There are so many diet books written every year. I find it amusing to watch as food fads come and go. Low fat, vegetarian, paleo, gluten free, raw, ketogenic, each year there is something new. I believe there is not one diet for everyone.

There are a few important things to consider here. Don't get stuck. I commonly see when someone starts eating well, they stay with the exact same diet and foods for a long time. An important idea to grasp is adaptability. In order to build health and maintain it, teaching our body to adapt to different circumstances is key. Also consider that shifting food contents and also shifting food macros at different times of year. A popular term for this is seasonally eating. For instance, the body can handle more sugar such as eating fruit in heat and sunshine vs. dark and cold winter times. This is primarily due to the mitochondria.

I believe something that deserves more attention is the bad fats. Bad fats, such as rancid oils or unstable oils, are one of the main reasons processed food is so detrimental to your health.

Back in the day, oils were very carefully protected by taking extreme cautions not to expose the oils to light. I urge you to stay away from certain oils such as canola oil, soybean oil and corn oil. If you were to look for a salad dressing in a grocery store, the vast majority of them contain one of these "bad" oils. Even the ones saying on the front "olive oil" will typically also have one of the bad oils mixed in with it.

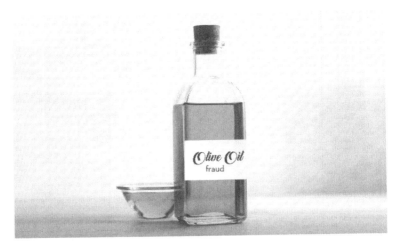

Consumer Reports found that only 9 out of 23 olive oils from California, Spain, and Italy passed as "extra virgin".[102] However, each of these olive oil brands claimed extra virgin certification on the label. A study conducted by the UC Davis Olive Center found that 69% of imported extra virgin olive oil (or EVOO) was not actually extra virgin.[103]

SO, HOW CAN YOU TELL THE DIFFERENCE?

Identifying Real Extra Virgin Olive Oil

Perhaps the most important step in avoiding poor-quality and tainted olive oil is being aware of the fraud in the marketplace. Unfortunately, just because a bottle claims to be "extra virgin", does not mean that it really is. While you can begin looking for brands that use the words "extra virgin" on the label, you may need to dig deeper to find the right quality of oil.

First things first, make sure you look for olive oil that is either "expeller-pressed", or "cold-pressed". You should also search for the following things when choosing authentic extra-virgin oil:[104]

- Price: If you want true extra-virgin olive oil, then you need to be prepared to pay for it. Any oil that's less than $10 per liter is unlikely to be the real thing. The numerous benefits of true extra-virgin olive oil are well-worth paying for. Olive oil that's truly extra-virgin tastes better, lasts longer, and comes with a host of vitality-boosting advantages.
- Certification: While you are checking the label for the "cold-pressed" production, look for a seal from the IOC. The International Olive Oil Council seal certifies the type of oil in the bottle.
- Dark glass: Dark glass not only looks more attractive on the store shelves, it also has a purpose for extra-virgin olive oil. Dark glass bottles prevent light from penetrating the bottle and damaging the fatty acids within. A bottle that's dark green, or black will limit oxidation and stop rancidity. Any oils that come in clear or plastic bottles should be avoided.
- Harvesting date: Check the label for a harvesting date to make sure that the oil is fresh. According to information from "The Olive Oil Times", stored away from light and heat, unopened bottles can last for two years. Once a bottle of extra-virgin

olive oil is open, it should be used within a few months. Additionally, true olive oil should be stored in cool, dark places.

- Consistency: Finally, keep in mind that a sign of a good product is one that solidifies when it is refrigerated or cold. The chemical structure of the fatty acids ensures this change in consistency. If you place your oil in the refrigerator, it should thicken and become cloudy. If the substance remains a liquid, then it is not true extra virgin olive oil.

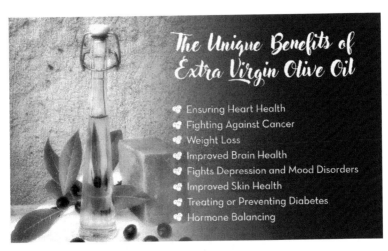

The Unique Benefits of Extra Virgin Olive Oil

- Ensuring Heart Health
- Fighting Against Cancer
- Weight Loss
- Improved Brain Health
- Fights Depression and Mood Disorders
- Improved Skin Health
- Treating or Preventing Diabetes
- Hormone Balancing

ALTERNATIVE COOKING OILS TO EVOO

High-quality extra-virgin olive oil is a fantastic option to have in your kitchen if you can avoid the fraudulent bottles. We covered above just some of the benefits that this delicious oil can give you when drizzled over foods and salads. However, that does not mean that it is the ideal option when it comes to cooking. There are some alternatives which can be far more effective, and beneficial for cooking, such as:

- Coconut oil: One of the best options for cooking, quality coconut oil is rich in lauric acid. Lauric acid is a form of saturated fat that helps to boost health HDL cholesterol. Coconut oil lowers cardiovascular risk, and it tastes great too.[105] Unlike fatty long-chain acids that are found in some oils, coconut oil is easier to digest. It's also anti-fungal and anti-microbial, and fully processed by the liver.
- Organic pastured butter: This substance, otherwise known as "Ghee", contains CLA and ALA which can promote weight loss. Additionally, these substances contain healthy short-chain fatty acids. They also come with a higher heat threshold, which make them ideal for cooking. Just remember to stick with organic only when you're purchasing any kind of butter.
- Avocado oil: Another great option for cooking, avocado oil is one of the only oils not derived from seeds or nuts. This oil has a fresh flavor that does not overpower delicate tastes with a high smoke point, which makes it ideal for browning, frying and more. Research also shows that avocado oil can fight back against the free radicals responsible for faster aging. Avocado oil is rich in mono-unsaturated fats. It also has heart-healthy omega-3, which can lower bad cholesterol called LDL cholesterol.[106]

- Red Palm Oil: Finally, red palm oil comes from the fruit of the palm, rather than the kernel. When unrefined, it's rich in beta-carotene, and vitamin E. Since it is stable under high heat, it is an ideal option for cooking.

Stay away from any food with a bad oil in it and watch your health increase! Bad oils are an extremely large cause today of a clogged lymphatic system!

Your genetics also play a role in what your diet should look like. Clinically, my team and I look at the genomics of each client to determine what foods are going to be best in the long term. It is important to note here that your current circumstances trump your genetics. Meaning, if you have genes that say you can digest the fat of dairy tolerant lactose, it is still possible that you have a dairy sensitivity and does not mean your genetics are "wrong". It most likely means you have parasites causing a dairy allergy or sensitivity.

Right now there are over 70 genes to look at alone for diet that allows us to determine what types of fats, the amount of carbs and the amount of protein that is best for you.

YOUR STRESS LEVELS

Consider your stressors and stress level as a factor in your healing. This not only includes physical stressors such as sitting at desk all day and chemical stressors such as toxic cologne or perfume you put on your body. A key area to consider is our mental and emotional stressors. Think of it as simply the state you are in is either helping or hurting you.

It is also relevant to talk about your past emotional traumas that have occurred. The more past emotional traumas there are, the tougher the case and more symptoms someone has. That shows me clinically that it plays a hugely important role in healing.

There are also experts in the field that believe Lyme disease shows up after a family reuniting and/or family resolution happens. I have seen instances where this does match up with individuals past timelines and situations.

CLOSING THOUGHTS

While it can seem overwhelming to consider all the other factors besides Lyme disease, it is also what gets chronic Lyme disease sufferers well. It simply comes down to identifying what are the source(s) to your health issues and in what order do they need to be addressed in. Do that and your health will improve so you can start living the life you want again!

Maximum Blessings,

Dr. Jay Davidson

ABOUT THE AUTHOR

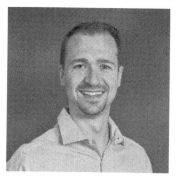

Dr. Jay Davidson focuses on functional, natural medicine. He is a husband and a father. He is also a popular speaker and a two time #1 international best-selling author. Dr. Jay was the host of the Chronic Lyme Disease Summit #1 and #2. He was also the host of the Parasite Summit and a co-host of The Detox Project, which had over 50,000 participants.

Dr. Jay Davidson is admired for his ability to bridge the gap between the scientific health community and the layperson. His holistic approach encompasses the mind, body and spirit. He works with his clients to formulate a simple, straightforward plan toward restoring health. This has gained him tremendous respect among the Lyme community and his colleagues.

Dr. Jay Davidson is an ambitious researcher and clinician in the health world. He is also the cofounder of Microbe Formulas.

Find out more at www.DrJayDavidson.com

CAN I ASK YOU FOR A FAVOR?

If you enjoyed this book, found it useful or otherwise then I'd really appreciate it if you would post a short review on Amazon. I do read all the reviews personally so that I can continually write what people are wanting.

Thanks for your support!

REFERENCES

1. Science: You Now Have a Shorter Attention Span Than a Goldfish. (n.d.). Retrieved September 06, 2017, from http://time.com/3858309/attention-spans-goldfish/
2. Meriläinen, L., Schwarzbach, A., Herranen, A., & Gilbert, L. (2015). Morphological and biochemical features of Borrelia burgdorferi pleomorphic forms. *Microbiology*, 161(3), 516-527. doi:10.1099/mic.0.000027 https://www.ncbi.nlm.nih.gov/pmc/articles/PMC4339653/
3. Teltow, G. J., Rawlings, J. A., & Fournier, P. V. (1991). Isolation of Borrelia burgdorferi from arthropods Collected in Texas. *The American Journal of Tropical Medicine and Hygiene*, 44(5), 469-474. doi:10.4269/ajtmh.1991.44.469 https://www.ncbi.nlm.nih.gov/pubmed/2063950
4. Anderson, J., Johnson, R., & Magnarelli, L. (1985). Identification of endemic foci of Lyme disease: isolation of Borrelia burgdorferi from feral rodents and ticks (Dermacentor variabilis). *Journal Clinical Microbiology*, 1, 36-38. https://www.ncbi.nlm.nih.gov/pubmed/3926816
5. Hynote, E. D., Mervine, P. C., & Stricker, R. B. (2012). Clinical evidence for rapid transmission of Lyme disease following a tickbite. *Diagnostic Microbiology and Infectious Disease*, 72(2), 188-192. doi:10.1016/j.diagmicrobio.2011.10.003 https://www.ncbi.nlm.nih.gov/pubmed/22104184
6. Vector Interactions and Molecular Adaptations of Lyme Disease and Relapsing Fever Spirochetes Associated with Transmission by Ticks - Volume 8, Number 2-February 2002 - Emerging Infectious Disease journal - CDC. (2010, July 14). Retrieved September 06, 2017, from https://wwwnc.cdc.gov/eid/article/8/2/01-0198_article
7. Cisak, Ewa E; Chmielewska, Jolanta J; Rajtar, Barbara B; Zwolinski, Jacek J; Jablonski, Leon L; Dutkiewicz, Jacek K. (2002) Study on the Occurrence of Borrelia Burgdorferi Sense Lato and Tick-Borne Encephalitis Virus (TBEV) in Ticks Collected in Lublin Region (Eastern Poland). *Annals of Agricultural and Environmental Medicine*, 9: 105-110. http://aaem.pl/abstracted.php?level=5&ICID=4513
8. Lyme Disease Transmitted by a Biting Fly. (1990). *New England Journal of Medicine, 322*(24), 1752-1752. doi:10.1056/nejm199006143222415 https://www.ncbi.nlm.nih.gov/pubmed/2342543
9. Doby JM; Chastel C; Couatarmanac'h A; Cousanca C; Chevrant-Breton J. (1985) Etiologic and epidemiologic questions posed by erythema chronicum migrans and Lyme disease. Apropos of 4 cases at the Regional Hospital Center, Rennes. *Bulletin de la Societe de pathoglogie exotique et de*

131

ses filiales, 78(4), 512-525.
https://www.ncbi.nlm.nih.gov/pubmed/4075471
10. Hubálek Z, Halouzka J, Juricová Z. (1998) Investigation of haematophagous arthropods for borreliae--summarized data, 1988-1996. *Folia Parasitologica*, 45(1):67-72.
https://www.ncbi.nlm.nih.gov/pubmed/9516997
11. Kampen, H., Schöler, A., Metzen, M., Oehme, R., Hartelt, K., Kimmig, P., & Maier, W. A. (2004). Neotrombicula autumnalis (Acari, Trombiculidae) as a vector for Borrelia burgdorferi S.L.? *Experimental and Applied Acarology, 33*(1/2), 93-102.
doi:10.1023/b:appa.0000029975.92510.90
https://www.ncbi.nlm.nih.gov/pubmed/15285141
12. Lopatina IuV, Vasil'eva IS, Gutova VP, Ershova AS, Burakova OV, Naumov RL, Petrova AD. (1999) [An experimental study of the capacity of the rat mite Ornithonyssus bacoti (Hirst, 1913) to ingest, maintain and transmit Borrelia]. *Meditsinskaia parazitologiia i parazitarnye bolezni*, Apr-Jun;(2):26-30.
https://www.ncbi.nlm.nih.gov/pubmed/10703202
13. Netušil, J., Zákovská, A., Horváth, R., Dendis, M., & Janouškovcová, E. (2005). Presence ofBorrelia burgdorferiSensu Lato in Mites Parasitizing Small Rodents. *Vector-Borne and Zoonotic Diseases, 5*(3), 227-232.
doi:10.1089/vbz.2005.5.227
https://www.ncbi.nlm.nih.gov/pubmed/16187890
14. Kosik-Bogacka, D. I., Kuźna-Grygiel, W., & Górnik, K. (2006). Borrelia burgdorferi sensu lato Infection in Mosquitoes from Szczecin Area. *Folia Biologica, 54*(1), 55-59.
doi:10.3409/173491606777919175
https://www.ncbi.nlm.nih.gov/pubmed/17044261
15. Zákovská A1, Nejedla P, Holíková A, Dendis M. (2002) Positive findings of Borrelia burgdorferi in Culex (Culex) pipiens pipiens larvae in the surrounding of Brno city determined by the PCR method. *Annals of agricultural and environmental medicine : AAEM.* 9(2):257-9.
https://www.ncbi.nlm.nih.gov/pubmed/12498597
16. Zákovská A1, Capková L, Serý O, Halouzka J, Dendis M. (2006) Isolation of Borrelia afzelii from overwintering Culex pipiens biotype molestus mosquitoes. *Annals of agricultural and environmental medicine : AAEM.* 13(2):345-8.
https://www.ncbi.nlm.nih.gov/pubmed/17199258
17. H., P., & H. (1998). Isolation of the spirochaete Borrelia afzelii from the mosquito Aedes vexans in the Czech Republic. *Medical and Veterinary Entomology, 12*(1), 103-105.
doi:10.1046/j.1365-2915.1998.00086.x
https://www.ncbi.nlm.nih.gov/pubmed/9513946

132

18. Halouzka, J., Wilske, B., Stünzner, D., Sanogo, Y., & Hubálek, Z. (1999). Isolation of Borrelia afzelii from Overwintering Culex pipiens Biotype molestus Mosquitoes. *Infection, 27*(4-5), 275-277. doi:10.1007/s150100050029 https://www.ncbi.nlm.nih.gov/pubmed/10885843
19. Kosik-Bogacka, D. I., Kuźna-Grygiel, W., & Jaborowska, M. (2007). Ticks and Mosquitoes as Vectors of *Borrelia burgdorferi s. l.* in the Forested Areas of Szczecin. *Folia Biologica, 55*(3), 143-146. doi:10.3409/173491607781492542 https://www.ncbi.nlm.nih.gov/pubmed/18274258
20. Teltow, G. J., Rawlings, J. A., & Fournier, P. V. (1991). Isolation of *Borrelia burgdorferi* from arthropods Collected in Texas. *The American Journal of Tropical Medicine and Hygiene, 44*(5), 469-474. doi:10.4269/ajtmh.1991.44.469 https://www.ncbi.nlm.nih.gov/pubmed/2063950
21. Pokorný P. (1989) [Incidence of the spirochete Borrelia burgdorferi in arthropods (Arthropoda) and antibodies in vertebrates (Vertebrata)]. *Ceskoslovenska epidemiologie, mikrobiologie, imunologie. Jan;38*(1):52-60. https://www.ncbi.nlm.nih.gov/pubmed/2646031
22. Magnarelli, L. A., Anderson, J. F., & Barbour, A. G. (1986). The Etiologic Agent of Lyme Disease in Deer Flies, Horse Flies, and Mosquitoes. *Journal of Infectious Diseases, 154*(2), 355-358. doi:10.1093/infdis/154.2.355 https://www.ncbi.nlm.nih.gov/pubmed/2873190
23. Magnarelli, L. A., Anderson, J. F. (1988) Ticks and biting insects infected with the etiologic agent of Lyme disease, Borrelia burgdorferi. *Journal of Clinical Microbiology, Aug;26*(8):1482-6. https://www.ncbi.nlm.nih.gov/pubmed/3170711
24. Burgess, EC. (1998) Borrelia Burgdorferi Infection in Wisconsin Horses and Cows. *Annals of the New York Academy of Sciences 539*(1): 235-43. www.ncbi.nlm.nih.gov/pubmed/3190095
25. Lyme Disease Facts -Lyme Facts. (n.d.). Retrieved September 06, 2017, from http://lymeandcancerservices.com/lyme/lyme-facts/
26. (2014) Possibility of Lyme Disease being Sexually Transmitted. In: Western Regional Meeting of the American Federation for Medical Research; 2014 Jan 25; Carmel, CA. *Journal of Investigative Medicine 62*(1): 280-81.
27. RECOVERY OF LYME SPIROCHETES BY PCR IN SEMEN SAMPLES OF PREVIOUSLY DIAGNOSED LYME DISEASE PATIENTS. (n.d.). Retrieved September 06, 2017, from http://whatislyme.com/recovery-of-lyme-spirochetes-by-pcr-in-semen-samples-of-previously-diagnosed-lyme-disease-patients/

28. Woodrum, J. E., & Oliver, J. H. (1999). Investigation of Venereal, Transplacental, and Contact Transmission of the Lyme Disease Spirochete, Borrelia burgdorferi, in Syrian Hamsters. *The Journal of Parasitology, 85*(3), 426. doi:10.2307/3285773
https://www.ncbi.nlm.nih.gov/pubmed/10386432
29. MacDonald AB. (1989) Gestational Lyme borreliosis. Implications for the fetus. *Rheumatic Diseases Clinics of North America. Nov;15*(4):657-77.
https://www.ncbi.nlm.nih.gov/pubmed/2685924
30. Sethi, S., Alcid, D., Kesarwala, H., & Tolan, R. W. (2009). Probable Congenital Babesiosis in Infant, New Jersey, USA. *Emerging Infectious Diseases, 15*(5), 788-791. doi:10.3201/eid1505.070808
https://www.ncbi.nlm.nih.gov/pmc/articles/PMC2687033/
31. Breitschwerdt, E. B., Maggi, R. G., Farmer, P., & Mascarelli, P. E. (2010). Molecular Evidence of Perinatal Transmission of Bartonella vinsonii subsp. berkhoffii and Bartonella henselae to a Child. *Journal of Clinical Microbiology, 48*(6), 2289-2293. doi:10.1128/jcm.00326-10
https://www.ncbi.nlm.nih.gov/pubmed/20392912
32. Nadelman, R., Sherer, C., Mack, L., Pavia, C., & Wormser, G. (1990). Survival of Borrelia burgdorferi in human blood stored under blood banking conditions. *Transfusion, 30*(4), 298-301. doi:10.1046/j.1537-2995.1990.30490273434.x
https://www.ncbi.nlm.nih.gov/pubmed/2349627
33. Klatt, Edward C. MD; Kumar, Vinay MBBS MD FRCPath. Robbins and Cotran Review of Pthology (Robbins Pathology), 4th Edition. Saunders; 2014 Oct 10.
34. Weintraub, P. (2013). *Cure unknown: inside the Lyme epidemic.* New York: St. Martins Griffin.
35. Stricker, R. B., & Phillips, S. E. (2003). Lyme disease without erythema migrans: cause for concern? *The American Journal of Medicine, 115*(1), 72-73. doi:10.1016/s0002-9343(03)00244-4 https://www.ncbi.nlm.nih.gov/pubmed/12867241
36. Centers for Disease Control and Prevention (CDC) (US). Lyme Disease - United Sates, 2001-2002. Morbidity and Morality Weekly Report (MMWR) [Internet]. 2004 May 7 [cited 2015 March 6]; 53(17): 365-69. Available from:
http://www.ncbi.nlm.nih.gov/pubmed/15129194
37. Stricker, Ray MD. The Treatment of Lyme Disease: A Medicolwegal Assessment. Expert Reviews in Anti-Infective Therapy. In: Lime Disease Association Conference (CALDA); 2014; California. [unpublished]
38. Centers for Disease Control and Prevention (US). Press Release Providing an Estimate of Americans Diagnoses with Lyme Disease Each Year. From: 2013 International

134

Conference on Lyme Borreliosis and Other Tick-Borne Diseases [Internet]. Boston, MA. 2013 Aug 19 https://www.cdc.gov/media/releases/2013/p0819-lyme-disease.html

39. LymeDiease.Org (formerly CALDA) (US). Sensitivity/Specificity of Commercial Two-Tier Testing for Lyme Disease. Table. CALDA; 2009. https://www.lymedisease.org/wp-content/uploads/2014/08/Image10-sensitivity.pdf

40. Ginsberg, H. S. (2008). Potential effects of mixed infections in ticks on transmission dynamics of pathogens: comparative analysis of published records. *Diseases of Mites and Ticks*, 29-41. doi:10.1007/978-1-4020-9695-2_5 https://www.ncbi.nlm.nih.gov/pubmed/18648996

41. Owen, D. C. (2006). Is Lyme disease always poly microbial? – The jigsaw hypothesis. *Medical Hypotheses, 67*(4), 860-864. doi:10.1016/j.mehy.2006.03.046 https://www.ncbi.nlm.nih.gov/pubmed/16814477

42. Buhner, Stephen Harrod. Healing Lyme: Natural Healing and Prevention of Lyme Borreliosis and Its Coinfections. Raven Press; 2005 Jun 25.

43. Horowitz, Richard I. MD. Why Can't I Get Better? Solving the Mystery of Lyme and Chronic Disease. St. Martin's Press; 2013 Nov 12.

44. Loo, C. S., Lam, N. S., Yu, D., Su, X., & Lu, F. (2017). Artemisinin and its derivatives in treating protozoan infections beyond malaria. *Pharmacological Research, 117*, 192-217. doi:10.1016/j.phrs.2016.11.012 https://www.ncbi.nlm.nih.gov/pubmed/27867026

45. Mary J. H, Aguilar-Delfin I, Telford III SR, Krause PJ, Persing DH. (2000) Babesiosis. *Clinical Microbiology Reviews* July vol. 13 no. 3 451-469. doi: 10.1128/CMR.13.3.451-469.2000 http://cmr.asm.org/content/13/3/451.full

46. Presented in: Integrated Lyme Solutions Conference; 2013 Jun 21-22; Dallas Texas. Academy of Comprehensive Integrative Medicine. [unpublished]

47. Sinha, Gunjan. What's Really Causing Gulf War Illness? One Man's Dogged Research Points to An Unusual (And likely) Suspect. Popular Science; 1999 Apr

48. Cohen, J. I. (2009). Optimal treatment for chronic active Epstein-Barr virus disease. *Pediatric Transplantation, 13*(4), 393-396. doi:10.1111/j.1399-3046.2008.01095.x https://www.ncbi.nlm.nih.gov/pmc/articles/PMC2776035/

49. Berris B. (1986) Chronic viral diseases. Canadian Medical Association Journal, Dec 1; 135(11): 1260–1268. https://www.ncbi.nlm.nih.gov/pmc/articles/PMC1491381/

50. Tunev, S. S., Hastey, C. J., Hodzic, E., Feng, S., Barthold, S. W., & Baumgarth, N. (2011). Lymphoadenopathy during Lyme Borreliosis Is Caused by Spirochete Migration-Induced Specific B Cell Activation. *PLoS Pathogens, 7*(5). doi:10.1371/journal.ppat.1002066 https://www.ncbi.nlm.nih.gov/pubmed/21637808

51. Kars, M., Yang, L., Gregor, M. F., Mohammed, B. S., Pietka, T. A., Finck, B. N., . . . Klein, S. (2010). Tauroursodeoxycholic Acid May Improve Liver and Muscle but Not Adipose Tissue Insulin Sensitivity in Obese Men and Women. *Diabetes, 59*(8), 1899-1905. doi:10.2337/db10-0308 https://www.ncbi.nlm.nih.gov/pmc/articles/PMC2911053/?tool= pmcentrez

52. Vettorazzi, J. F., Ribeiro, R. A., Borck, P. C., Branco, R. C., Soriano, S., Merino, B., . . . Carneiro, E. M. (2016). The bile acid TUDCA increases glucose-induced insulin secretion via the cAMP/PKA pathway in pancreatic beta cells. *Metabolism, 65*(3), 54-63. doi:10.1016/j.metabol.2015.10.021 https://www.ncbi.nlm.nih.gov/pubmed/26892516

53. Mosbah, I. B., Alfany-Fernández, I., Martel, C., Zaouali, M. A., Bintanel-Morcillo, M., Rimola, A., . . . Peralta, C. (2010). Endoplasmic reticulum stress inhibition protects steatotic and non-steatotic livers in partial hepatectomy under ischemia–reperfusion. *Cell Death and Disease, 1*(7). doi:10.1038/cddis.2010.29 http://www.nature.com/cddis/journal/v1/n7/full/cddis201029a.ht ml?foxtrotcallback=true

54. https://www.researchgate.net/profile/Xiao_Li_Pan/publication/2 36206558_Efficacy_and_safety_of_tauroursodeoxycholic_acid _in_the_treatment_of_liver_cirrhosis_A_double-blind_randomized_controlled_trial/links/585b923108ae8fce48f a6cff.pdf

55. Vang, S., Longley, K., Steer, C. J., & Low, W. C. (2014). The Unexpected Uses of Urso- and Tauroursodeoxycholic Acid in the Treatment of Non-liver Diseases. *Global Advances in Health and Medicine, 3*(3), 58-69. doi:10.7453/gahmj.2014.017 https://www.ncbi.nlm.nih.gov/pmc/articles/PMC4030606/

56. Bautista-Toledo, I., Ferro-García, M. A., Rivera-Utrilla, J., Moreno-Castilla, C., & Fernández, F. J. (2005). Bisphenol A Removal from Water by Activated Carbon. Effects of Carbon Characteristics and Solution Chemistry. *Environmental Science & Technology, 39*(16), 6246-6250. doi:10.1021/es0481169 http://pubs.acs.org/doi/abs/10.1021/es0481169

57. Decker WJ, Corby DG. (1980) Activated charcoal adsorbs aflatoxin B1. *Veterinary and Human*

Toxicology. Dec;22(6):388-9.
https://www.ncbi.nlm.nih.gov/pubmed/6782748
58. Bautista-Toledo, I., Ferro-García, M. A., Rivera-Utrilla, J., Moreno-Castilla, C., & Fernández, F. J. (2005). Bisphenol A Removal from Water by Activated Carbon. Effects of Carbon Characteristics and Solution Chemistry. *Environmental Science & Technology, 39*(16), 6246-6250. doi:10.1021/es0481169
http://pubs.acs.org/doi/abs/10.1021/es0481169
59. Hultén, B., Heath, A., Mellstrand, T., & Hedner, T. (1986). Does Alcohol Absorb to Activated Charcoal? *Human Toxicology, 5*(3), 211-212. doi:10.1177/096032718600500311
https://www.ncbi.nlm.nih.gov/pubmed/3710499
60. First Aiders Guide to Alcohol. (n.d.). Retrieved September 06, 2017, from http://www.princeton.edu/~oa/safety/alcohol.shtml
61. Jain, N. K. (1986). Activated Charcoal, Simethicone, and Intestinal Gas: A Double-Blind Study. *Annals of Internal Medicine, 105*(1), 61. doi:10.7326/0003-4819-105-1-61
https://www.ncbi.nlm.nih.gov/pubmed/3521259
62. Hoekstra, J., & Erkelens, D. (1987). Effect Of Activated Charcoal On Hypercholesterolaemia. *The Lancet, 330*(8556), 455. doi:10.1016/s0140-6736(87)90990-1
https://www.ncbi.nlm.nih.gov/pubmed/2874369
63. Maizels, R. M., Mcsorley, H. J., & Smyth, D. J. (2014). Helminths in the hygiene hypothesis: sooner or later? *Clinical & Experimental Immunology, 177*(1), 38-46. doi:10.1111/cei.12353
https://www.ncbi.nlm.nih.gov/pubmed/24749722
64. Mathison, B. A., & Pritt, B. S. (2014). Laboratory Identification of Arthropod Ectoparasites. *Clinical Microbiology Reviews, 27*(1), 48-67. doi:10.1128/cmr.00008-13
https://www.ncbi.nlm.nih.gov/pmc/articles/PMC3910909/
65. Group, P. C. (2016, May 19). Lyme Bacteria Hides Inside Parasitic Worms, Causing Chronic Brain Diseases. Retrieved September 06, 2017, from http://www.prnewswire.com/news-releases/lyme-bacteria-hides-inside-parasitic-worms-causing-chronic-brain-diseases-300270742.html
66. Parasitic Infections also occur in the United States. (n.d.). Retrieved September 06, 2017, from https://www.cdc.gov/media/releases/2014/p0508-npi.html
67. Fecal Matter Found on 72 Percent of Grocery Carts. (n.d.). Retrieved September 06, 2017, from http://www.foxnews.com/health/2011/03/03/fecal-matter-72-percent-grocery-carts.html
68. Astagneau, E. D., Hadengue, A., Degott, C., Vilgrain, V., Erlinger, S., & Benhamou, J. P. (1994). Biliary obstruction resulting from Strongyloides **stercoralis** infection. Report of a

137

case. *Gut, 35*(5), 705-706. doi:10.1136/gut.35.5.705
https://www.ncbi.nlm.nih.gov/pmc/articles/PMC1374762/pdf/gu
t00539-0141.pdf
69. Sotto A, Gra B. (1985) Hepatic manifestations in
    giardiasis. *Acta Gastroenterologica Latinoamericana,15*(2):89-
    94. https://www.ncbi.nlm.nih.gov/pubmed/3835766
70. Das, A. (2014). Hepatic and biliary ascariasis. *Journal of
    Global Infectious Diseases, 6*(2), 65. doi:10.4103/0974-
    777x.132042
    https://www.ncbi.nlm.nih.gov/pmc/articles/PMC4049042/
71. Walker, M. D., & Zunt, J. R. (2005). Neuroparasitic Infections:
    Cestodes, Trematodes, and Protozoans. *Seminars in
    Neurology, 25*(03), 262-277. doi:10.1055/s-2005-917663
    https://www.ncbi.nlm.nih.gov/pmc/articles/PMC2683840/
72. Halliez, M. C. (2013). Extra-intestinal and long term
    consequences of Giardia duodenalis infections. *World Journal
    of Gastroenterology, 19*(47), 8974.
    doi:10.3748/wjg.v19.i47.8974
    https://www.ncbi.nlm.nih.gov/pmc/articles/PMC3870550/
73. Bagi, M. A. (n.d.). Imaging of Parasitic Diseases of the
    Gastrointestinal Tract. *Imaging of Parasitic Diseases*, 73-102.
    doi:10.1007/978-3-540-49354-9_4
    https://www.ncbi.nlm.nih.gov/pubmed/16582677
74. Kavet, R. (1996). EMF and current cancer
    concepts. *Bioelectromagnetics, 17*(5), 339-357.
    doi:10.1002/(sici)1521-186x(1996)17:5<339::aid-
    bem1>3.0.co;2-4
    https://www.ncbi.nlm.nih.gov/pubmed/8915543
75. Murphy, G. (2009). Ultraviolet radiation and
    immunosuppression. *British Journal of Dermatology, 161*, 90-
    95. doi:10.1111/j.1365-2133.2009.09455.x
    https://www.ncbi.nlm.nih.gov/pubmed/19775363
76. Verma, S., & Gupta, M. L. (2015). Radiation-induced
    hematopoietic myelosuppression and genotoxicity get
    significantly countered by active
    principles ofPodophyllum hexandrum: A study in strain 'A'
    mice. *International Journal of Radiation Biology, 91*(9), 757-
    770. doi:10.3109/09553002.2015.1062576
    https://www.ncbi.nlm.nih.gov/pubmed/26073527
77. Maloney, E. L. (2016). Controversies in Persistent (Chronic)
    Lyme Disease. *Journal of Infusion Nursing, 39*(6), 369-375.
    doi:10.1097/nan.0000000000000195
    https://www.ncbi.nlm.nih.gov/pmc/articles/PMC5102277/
78. Stratton, J. A., Byfield, P. E., Byfield, J. E., Small, R. C.,
    Benfield, J., & Pilch, Y. (1975). A comparison of the acute
    effects of radiation therapy, including or excluding the thymus,
    on the lymphocyte subpopulations of cancer patients. *Journal*

of Clinical Investigation, 56(1), 88-97. doi:10.1172/jci108084
https://www.ncbi.nlm.nih.gov/pubmed/1095613
79. Abdelhalim MA, Al-Ayed MS, Moussa SA, Abd Al-Sheri Ael-H. (2015) The effects of gamma-radiation on red blood cell corpuscles and dimensional properties in rats. *Pakistan Journal of Pharmaceutical Sciences*, Sep;28(5 Suppl):1819-22. https://www.ncbi.nlm.nih.gov/pubmed/26525021
80. Wood, A. W. (2006). How dangerous are mobile phones, transmission masts, and electricity pylons? *Archives of Disease in Childhood, 91*(4), 361-366. doi:10.1136/adc.2005.072561 https://www.ncbi.nlm.nih.gov/pmc/articles/PMC2065971/
81. Peer-reviewed scientific studies on EMF related subjects. (n.d.). Retrieved September 06, 2017, from http://www.powerwatch.org.uk/science/studies.asp
82. Ross, C. L., Siriwardane, M., Almeida-Porada, G., Porada, C. D., Brink, P., Christ, G. J., & Harrison, B. S. (2015). The effect of low-frequency electromagnetic field on human bone marrow stem/progenitor cell differentiation. *Stem Cell Research, 15*(1), 96-108. doi:10.1016/j.scr.2015.04.009 https://www.ncbi.nlm.nih.gov/pmc/articles/PMC4516580/
83. P. (2017, July 02). Hazards of EMFs and RF Microwave Radiation. Retrieved September 06, 2017, from http://scientists4wiredtech.com/2017/03/rfr-hazards/
84. Electromagnetic fields and public health. (n.d.). Retrieved September 06, 2017, from http://www.who.int/peh-emf/publications/facts/fs296/en/
85. Ma, A. (2015, June 29). A Sad Number Of Americans Sleep With Their Smartphone In Their Hand. Retrieved September 06, 2017, from http://www.huffingtonpost.com/2015/06/29/smartphone-behavior-2015_n_7690448.html
86. Gharib, O. A. (2014). Effect of kombucha on some trace element levels in different organs of electromagnetic field exposed rats. *Journal of Radiation Research and Applied Sciences, 7*(1), 18-22. doi:10.1016/j.jrras.2013.11.002 http://www.sciencedirect.com/science/article/pii/S16878507130 00149
87. Vīna, I., Semjonovs, P., Linde, R., & Deniņa, I. (2014). Current Evidence on Physiological Activity and Expected Health Effects of Kombucha Fermented Beverage. *Journal of Medicinal Food, 17*(2), 179-188. doi:10.1089/jmf.2013.0031 https://www.ncbi.nlm.nih.gov/pubmed/24192111
88. Berek, L., Petri, I., Mesterházy, Á, Téren, J., & Molnár, J. (2001). Effects of mycotoxins on human immune functions in vitro. *Toxicology in Vitro, 15*(1), 25-30. doi:10.1016/s0887-

2333(00)00055-2
https://www.ncbi.nlm.nih.gov/pubmed/11259866
89. Is toxic mold standing in the way of your Lyme recovery?
(2017, March 28). Retrieved September 06, 2017, from
https://www.lymedisease.org/toxic-mold-standing-way-lyme-
recovery/
90. Retrieved September 06, 2017, from
http://health.mo.gov/living/environment/indoorair/mold.php
91. Brewer, J., Thrasher, J., & Hooper, D. (2013). Chronic Illness
Associated with Mold and Mycotoxins: Is Naso-Sinus Fungal
Biofilm the Culprit? *Toxins, 6*(1), 66-80.
doi:10.3390/toxins6010066
https://www.ncbi.nlm.nih.gov/pmc/articles/PMC3920250/
92. Jarvis, B. B., Zhou, Y., Jiang, J., Wang, S., Sorenson, W. G.,
Hintikka, E., . . . Dearborn, D. G. (1996). Toxigenic Molds in
Water-Damaged Buildings: Dechlorogriseofulvins from
Memnoniella echinata. *Journal of Natural Products, 59*(6), 553-
554. doi:10.1021/np960395t
https://www.ncbi.nlm.nih.gov/pubmed/8786360
93. Visagie C.M., Houbraken J., Frisvad J.C., Hong S.-B.,
Klaassen C.H.W.,Perrone G., et al. (2014) Identification and
nomenclature of the genus Penicillium. *Studies in Mycology*,
Jun; 78: 343–371.
https://www.ncbi.nlm.nih.gov/pmc/articles/PMC4261876/
94. Sosa EE, Cohen PR, Tschen JA. (2012) Cladosporium scalp
infection. *Skinmed*, Nov-Dec;10(6):393-4.
https://www.ncbi.nlm.nih.gov/pubmed/23346670
95. Granja, L. Z., Pinto, L., Almeida, C. A., Alviano, D. S., Silva, M.
H., Ejzemberg, R., & Alviano, C. S. (2009). Spores of
Mucor ramosissimus, Mucor plumbeus and
Mucor circinelloides and their ability to activate human
complement system in vitro. *Medical Mycology*, 1-7.
doi:10.1080/13693780903096669
https://www.ncbi.nlm.nih.gov/pubmed/20141371
96. Implementing Health-Protective Features and Practices in
Buildings: Workshop Proceedings: Federal Facilities Council
Technical Report #148 (No. 148) by National Research Council
97. http://www.gov.scot/Resource/Doc/156479/0042008.pdf
98. Mohamed E.Zain (2011) Impact of mycotoxins on humans and
animals. *Journal of Saudi Chemical Society, 15*(2), April, 129-
144. https://doi.org/10.1016/j.jscs.2010.06.006
http://www.sciencedirect.com/science/article/pii/S13196103100
00827
99. Bennett J. W., Klich M. (2003) Mycotoxins. *Clinical
Microbiology Reviews.* Jul; 16(3): 497–516.
doi: 10.1128/CMR.16.3.497-516.2003
https://www.ncbi.nlm.nih.gov/pmc/articles/PMC164220/

100. UNITED STATES DEPARTMENT OF LABOR. (n.d.). Retrieved September 06, 2017, from https://www.osha.gov/dts/shib/shib101003.html
101. A Brief Guide to Mold, Moisture and Your Home. (2017, February 21). Retrieved September 06, 2017, from https://www.epa.gov/mold/brief-guide-mold-moisture-and-your-home
102. How to Find the Best Extra-Virgin Olive Oil. (n.d.). Retrieved September 06, 2017, from https://www.consumerreports.org/cro/magazine/2012/09/how-to-find-the-best-extra-virgin-olive-oil/index.htm
103. http://olivecenter.ucdavis.edu/publications/olive%20oil%20final%20071410%20updated.pdf
104. Karunathilaka, S. R., Kia, A. F., Srigley, C., Chung, J. K., & Mossoba, M. M. (2016). Nontargeted, Rapid Screening of Extra Virgin Olive Oil Products for Authenticity Using Near-Infrared Spectroscopy in Combination with Conformity Index and Multivariate Statistical Analyses. *Journal of Food Science, 81*(10). doi:10.1111/1750-3841.13432 https://www.ncbi.nlm.nih.gov/pubmed/27626761
105. Eyres, L., Eyres, M. F., Chisholm, A., & Brown, R. C. (2016). Coconut oil consumption and cardiovascular risk factors in humans. *Nutrition Reviews, 74*(4), 267-280. doi:10.1093/nutrit/nuw002 https://www.ncbi.nlm.nih.gov/pubmed/26946252
106. Carvajal-Zarrabal, O., Nolasco-Hipolito, C., Aguilar-Uscanga, M. G., Melo-Santiesteban, G., Hayward-Jones, P. M., & Barradas-Dermitz, D. M. (2014). Avocado Oil Supplementation Modifies Cardiovascular Risk Profile Markers in a Rat Model of Sucrose-Induced Metabolic Changes. *Disease Markers*, 2014, 1-8. doi:10.1155/2014/386425 https://www.ncbi.nlm.nih.gov/pmc/articles/PMC3955619/

Made in the USA
Lexington, KY
14 June 2018